Dx/Rx:

Cervical Cancer
An Approach to Preinvasive and Invasive Malignancies of the Cervix

Don S. Dizon, MD, FACP

Program in Women's Oncology,
Women & Infants' Hospital
Warren Alpert Medical School of Brown University
Providence, RI

Katina Robison, MD

Program in Women's Oncology,
Women & Infants' Hospital
Warren Alpert Medical School of Brown University
Providence, RI

Series Editor: Manish A. Shah, MD

Micrographs courtesy of Margaret M. Steinhoff, MD, Department of Pathology, Women & Infants' Hospital, The Warren Alpert Medical School of Brown University, Providence, RI

JONES AND BARTLETT PUBLISHERS
Sudbury, Massachusetts
BOSTON   TORONTO   LONDON   SINGAPORE

World Headquarters
Jones and Bartlett Publishers
40 Tall Pine Drive
Sudbury, MA 01776
978-443-5000
info@jbpub.com
www.jbpub.com

Jones and Bartlett Publishers Canada
6339 Ormindale Way
Mississauga, Ontario L5V 1J2
Canada

Jones and Bartlett Publishers International
Barb House, Barb Mews
London W6 7PA
United Kingdom

Jones and Bartlett's books and products are available through most bookstores and online booksellers. To contact Jones and Bartlett Publishers directly, call 800-832-0034, fax 978-443-8000, or visit our website, www.jbpub.com.

Substantial discounts on bulk quantities of Jones and Bartlett's publications are available to corporations, professional associations, and other qualified organizations. For details and specific discount information, contact the special sales department at Jones and Bartlett via the above contact information or send an email to specialsales@jbpub.com.

The authors, editor, and publisher have made every effort to provide accurate information. However, they are not responsible for errors, omissions, or for any outcomes related to the use of the contents of this book and take no responsibility for the use of the products and procedures described. Treatments and side effects described in this book may not be applicable to all people; likewise, some people may require a dose or experience a side effect that is not described herein. Drugs and medical devices are discussed that may have limited availability controlled by the Food and Drug Administration (FDA) for use only in a research study or clinical trial. Research, clinical practice, and government regulations often change the accepted standard in this field. When consideration is being given to use of any drug in the clinical setting, the health care provider or reader is responsible for determining FDA status of the drug, reading the package insert, and reviewing prescribing information for the most up-to-date recommendations on dose, precautions, and contraindications, and determining the appropriate usage for the product. This is especially important in the case of drugs that are new or seldom used.

Library of Congress Cataloging-in-Publication Data
Dizon, Don S.
  Dx/Rx. Cervical cancer / Don S. Dizon, Katina Robison.
    p. ; cm. — (Jones and Bartlett publishers Dx/Rx oncology series)
  Includes bibliographical references and index.
  ISBN-13: 978-0-7637-5348-1
  ISBN-10: 0-7637-5348-3
  1. Cervix uteri—Cancer—Handbooks, manuals, etc. I. Robison, Katina. II. Title.
III. Title: Cervical cancer. IV. Series.
  [DNLM: 1. Uterine Cervical Neoplasms—Handbooks. WP 39 D622d 2008]
  RC280.U8D59 2008
  616.99'446—dc22
  6048   2007017089

Production Credits
Executive Publisher: Christopher Davis
Production Director: Amy Rose
Associate Editor: Kathy Richardson
Production Editor: Daniel Stone
Marketing Associate: Rebecca Wasley
V.P., Manufacturing and Inventory Control:
  Therese Connell

Composition: ATLIS Graphics
Cover Design: Anne Spencer
Printing and Binding: Malloy, Inc.
Cover Printing: Malloy, Inc.

Printed in the United States of America
11 10 09 08 07   10 9 8 7 6 5 4 3 2 1

Contents

Preface

Thankfully cervical cancer is not a common cancer in the United States. This fact stands as a testament to the benefits of a widely accepted screening test: the Pap smear. With Pap smears, most cervical lesions are being caught early, even before they become cancer; as a consequence, this disease does not affect or interfere with the lives of most women. Of course, there are still women being diagnosed with advanced disease—those who have to undergo more complicated therapies including chemotherapy and radiation, and are even faced with the prospects of radical surgery. But for the vast majority of women screened with Pap smears, this fate can be avoided; estimates show a steady decline in the death rates from cervical cancer by 4% a year. Although cervical cancer will represent fewer than 12,000 cases in the United States, more than 400,000 women will be diagnosed internationally, with the majority diagnosed in less-developed regions. So for the rest of the world, cervical cancer continues to be a major health problem.

DxRx Cervical Cancer has been designed as a comprehensive handbook for the treatments of both preinvasive and invasive cervical pathology. Our aim is to provide an overview of the problem and the clinical approach to it, which can be accessible both nationally and internationally. It comes at a time of great change and hope for women with cervical cancer and for those who wish to avoid it. Within this book we bring the messages of early detection and screening alongside the breakthroughs in cancer management including surgical techniques and the increased use of definitive chemoradiation. Finally, it brings the message of prevention and the hope of cervical cancer vaccines, which have the potential to greatly reduce, if not eradicate, this disease in the future.

I would like to thank Chris Davis and Kathy Richardson at Jones & Bartlett for this wonderful opportunity, and Katina Robison, for rising to the challenge with me. In addition, I dedicate this book to my partner, Henry, and our daughter, Isabelle; my mom and dad, Marilyn Stoll, Michelle and Mel Ramos, Mae Dizon, Precy and Ben Goldstein, and to Marie, Ed, Stella, and Jude Sablan. I would also like to dedicate this book to my colleagues at the Program in Women's Oncology and to my "old" family at Memorial Sloan-Kettering Cancer Center, especially to David R. Spriggs, whose friendship and mentoring I am forever grateful for. Lastly, I dedicate this book to those women with cervical cancer whom I have been honored to care for, listen to, and learn from.

Don S. Dizon, MD FACP

Epidemiology, Risk Factors, and Co-factors

■ Epidemiology

- Cervical cancer and preinvasive cervical neoplasia are significant problems both in the United States and worldwide.
- Eighty-three percent of cervical cancer cases occur in developing countries.
  - In 2006, 510,000 women were diagnosed with cervical cancer and 288,000 cervical cancer related deaths occurred.[1,3]
  - Highest incidence rates are observed in sub-Saharan Africa, Melanesia, Latin America and the Caribbean, southcentral Asia and southeast Asia.
- In the United States it is the seventh most frequent cancer diagnosed in women with an estimated 11,150 women diagnosed with invasive cervical cancer in 2007 and approximately 3,670 deaths from cervical cancer.[1,2]
  - Between 1955 and 1992, the death rate from cervical cancer in American women has decreased by 74%, which has been attributed to widespread screening using the Papanicolaou (Pap) test.
  - The death rate continues to decline by 4% per year.[2]
- Fifty percent of cases are diagnosed between the ages of 35 and 55 years. It rarely occurs under the age of 20 years, but approximately 20% of women are diagnosed after the age of 65.
- Racial Demographics
  - Incidence rates of invasive cervical cancer vary among racial groups, with Hispanic women having the highest incidence rates, followed by African-American women. Caucasian, Asian, Pacific Islander and Non-Hispanic White women all have the lowest incidence rates.

- Hispanic women are more likely than Caucasian women to develop invasive cervical cancer, with rates increasing substantially after age 40.
- African-American women have significantly higher incident rates after age 50 and have the highest cervical cancer mortality.[3]

■ Risk Factors and Co-Factors

- There are many demographic and behavioral risk factors associated with persistent oncogenic infection and for cervical cancer. There are also important co-factors that are associated with an increased risk of cervical cancer.[4]
- Human Papillomavirus (HPV)
  - Infection with this oncogenic virus is considered the major biologic risk factor for developing precancerous lesions and invasive cancer of the cervix.
  - Virtually all cervical cancers are causally related to HPV infection
  - HPV types are classified by their risk of being oncogenic, as high-risk and low-risk.[5] See Table 1-1.
  - While HPV infection is a "necessary" precursor for the development of cervical cancer, the vast majority of women will not develop cervical cancer, strongly suggesting it is not "sufficient" and that other factors play a role in cervical carcinogenesis.[6]
  - Incidence and Prevalence
    - 20 million people in the U.S. are currently infected by HPV.
    - Approximately half are in those aged 15 to 25 years.
    - It is estimated that up to 80% of sexually active women will be infected by age 50.[7]

Table 1-1:   Human Papillomavirus Subtypes

High-risk types: 16, 18, 31, 33, 35, 39, 45, 51, 52, 56, 58, 59, 68, 73, 82
Low-risk types: 6, 11, 40, 42, 43, 44, 54, 61, 70, 72, 81, CP6108
Potentially high-risk types: 26, 53, 66

Adapted from reference 15.

- Transmission of HPV
  - Genital HPV is usually transmitted via vaginal (or anal) intercourse, though any form of sexual activity can result in HPV infection.
  - There is some debate about the risk of transmission of HPV from non-sexual activity, however multiple epidemiologic studies have suggested that intravaginal HPV infection does not occur in virginal or non-sexually active girls/women.[8–11]
  - More than 50% of college-age women acquired HPV infection within 4 years of fist intercourse.
  - Vertical transmission from mother to newborn is uncommon.[3,12]
  - HPV is exclusively an intraepithelial microbe and grows in the basal epithelial cells of the cervix.[24]
  - Microtrauma increases the likelihood of infection of the cervical epithelium.[25,26]
- Biology of the Human Papillomavirus
  - Papillomaviruses are small, double-stranded, circular DNA viruses that infect epithelial tissues.
  - More than 100 types of HPV described. Of these only 14 have been classified as oncogenic.
  - Genomes are organized into an early, a late, and a long control region (Figure 1).
    - The early control region contains genes E6 and E7 are essential in the HPV-induced processes of cellular transformation and immortalization.
    - The late control region contains genes L1 and L2 encode the viral capsid proteins.
- Mechanism of neoplastic transformation in cervical cells by HPV
  - High-risk HPV-types are associated with 97% of cervical carcinomas.
  - The viral genome is integrated into host cell chromosomes in cervical epithelial cells. Those cells with integrated HPV genes multiply faster which may be due to the increased expression of oncoproteins E6 and E7, which respectively bind and inactivate tumor suppressor proteins p53 and pRB.
  - Chromosomal instability has also been shown to occur in epithelial cells expressing E6 and E7 oncogenes from high-risk HPV.[5]

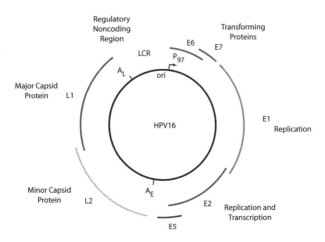

Figure 1-1: The human papillomavirus (HPV) genome.

- 500,000 high-grade cervical intraepithelial neoplasia (CIN) lesions are diagnosed each year in the U.S. and about 50% to 60% are attributable to HPV 16 and HPV 18
- Cervical intraepithelial neoplasia (CIN) is caused by both high-risk and low-risk HPV types.
  - 25% by either HPV 16 and HPV 18
- 70% of invasive cervical cancers in the U.S. are caused by HPV types 16 and 18
  - HPV 18 is more commonly detected (30%) in adenocarcinoma of the cervix than in squamous cell carcinoma (10 to 15%).
- Most HPV infections are transient and resolve within a year or two.[3,13] Refer to Table 1-2.
  - Approximately 90% of *low-grade lesions* in adolescents resolve without treatment.
  - The development of invasive cancer from HPV acquisition takes 20 years on average[3]
- The time from high-grade lesions to invasive cancer is the longest amount of time.
- HPV can become persistent by avoiding the immune system through multiple mechanisms:
  - It infects and multiplies in keratinocytes, which have a naturally short lifespan. As a result, HPV

Table 1-2:   Natural History of Cervical Intraepithelial Lesions (CIN)

	Regress	Persist	Progress to CIS	Progress to invasion
CIN 1	57%	32%	11%	1%
CIN2	43%	35%	22%	5%
CIN3	32%	56%	—	>12%

Adapted from reference 16.

does not need to destroy the host cell and therefore, does not trigger apoptosis-induced inflammation or immune response.[24,26]

- HPV results in the downregulation of interferon genes, which have antiviral and antiproliferative properties.[27,28]
- HPV oncoproteins, E6 and E7 can directly inhibit antiviral pathways in cells.[29,30]

- Following natural HPV infection, detectable HPV antibody levels are seen only in 50% of women, and even then, it is present in low titers. Low levels may not confer protection against future HPV infection.[24,31]

- Antibodies to HPV have not been shown to protect against ongoing infection.[32]

- Human Immunodeficiency Virus
  - Immunosuppresion has been a recognized risk factor for cervical cancer for many years.
  - The relationship between HIV infection and abnormal cervical cytology was first described in 1987.[14] HIV-infected women develop cervical carcinoma-in-situ lesions at younger ages (32.7 years) compared to non-HIV-infected women (47.5 years). In addition, the interval for developing invasive disease is shorter in HIV-infected women (3.2 versus 15.7 years).
  - In 1993, the Centers for Disease Control and Prevention (CDC) designated moderate and severe cervical dysplasia as early symptomatic HIV infection.

Invasive cervical cancer was designated as an AIDS-defining condition.

- A large trial, the Women's Interagency HIV Study (WIHS), found that 40% of HIV-infected women have abnormal Papanicolaou's (Pap) smears compared to only 17% among non-HIV-infected controls.
  - The majority of abnormal Pap smears are low-grade lesions.
- There are many variables impacting the risk for cervical disease in HIV-infected women, including:
  - Infection with HPV
    - Prevalence rate up to 95% in HIV-infected women
  - CD4 count
    - 40.5% of women with CD4 counts <200 and low-grade SIL (LGSIL) developed high-grade SIL (HGSIL) within 12 months.
    - In women with CD4 counts >500 and LGSIL, HGSIL did not develop.[14]
  - HIV viral load
    - The median viral load in a study of HIV-infected women in South Africa with abnormal cervical cytology was 30,000-40,000 compared to 11,500 in non-HIV-infected women.[15]
  - Type of HIV infection (HIV-1 versus HIV-2)
  - Highly active antiretroviral therapy (HAART)
- HIV-infection may interact with HPV in ways other than suppressing the immune system.
  - HIV modulates cytokine expression, which may alter HPV regulation.
  - HIV has been shown to up-regulate HPV expression through the 'tat' gene in *in vitro* studies.[14]
- Demographic factors
  - Age
    - Rates of invasive cervical cancer rise with age in all racial groups except Caucasian.[16]
  - Race
  - Socioeconomic status

- ■ Increased rates of cervical cancer are seen among women of lower socioeconomic status.
- • Education level
  - ■ Women with less than high school education have an increased risk of cervical cancer.[17]
- ■ Behavioral factors
  - • While all sexually active women are at risk for cervical cancer, a number of factors are associated with an increased risk of cervical cancer:
    - ■ Number of sexual partners: the greater the number of sexual partners the greater the risk of cervical cancer due to the increased risk of exposure to the Human Papilloma Virus (HPV).[18,19]
    - ■ Age of first intercourse: Age less than 18 years at first intercourse is associated with a two-fold increased risk of developing cervical cancer.
    - ■ Early age at first pregnancy: Age less than 20 years at the time of first birth is associated with over a two-fold increased risk of developing cervical cancer.
    - ■ History of sexually transmitted infections
  - • Multiparity
    - ■ The risk of cervical cancer increases with the increase in number of full-term pregnancies.[18]
  - • Cigarette Smoking
    - ■ There is a positive relationship between cigarette smoking and the development of cervical cancer.[4]
      - • Cigarette smoking appears to increase the risk of development of squamous cell carcinoma of the cervix, but does not play a role in the development of adenocarcinoma of the cervix.[16]
      - • Smoking cessation and/or reduction has been shown to decrease the cervical lesion size.[20]
      - • A history of cigarette smoking does not appear to increase the risk of cervical cancer.[18] However, the length of cigarette smoke exposure may have an impact on developing cervical dysplasia.
      - • Women exposed to second hand smoke have approximately a two-fold increased risk of developing cervical dysplasia.[19]

- Several mechanisms have been postulated to account for the association between cervical cancer and cigarette smoking.
  - There is secretion of cigarette smoke by-products, including nicotine, in cervical mucus of tobacco users. DNA adducts are more common in cervical epithelium of smokers. Cigarette smoke by-products may have a direct mutagenic effect on the cervical epithelium.[4]
  - In smokers, there is a reduction in the number of Langerhans cells in the cervices compared to nonsmokers. This reduction may result in decreased local immunity, leading to increased HPV susceptibility.[21]
- Hormones
  - The relationship between oral contraception (OCP) use and the development of cervical cancer remains controversial. It has been difficult to control for the fact that women using oral contraceptives tend to not use other barrier contraceptives and have more sexual contacts.
    - A recent meta-analysis concluded the relative risk of cervical cancer among women using oral contraceptives for 5 to 9 years is 1.6 and for greater than 10 years is 2.2.[4]
    - In the Women's Health Initiative, use of estrogen plus progestin was associated with increased cervical dysplasia, but had no impact on the incidence of cervical cancer.[22]
    - Other studies have suggested a shorter timd to onset of high-grade lesions and cervical cancer in OCP users.[4,23]
  - Diethylstilbestrol (DES)
    - DES is a synthetic non-steroidal estrogen that was used in the 1970s to prevent early pregnancy loss.[7] It was listed as a carcinogen in 1985.
    - There is a strong association between in utero DES exposure and both vaginal and cervical clear cell adenocarcinoma.[7]

- Dietary Factors
  - There is inconclusive evidence on the relationship between cervical cancer and diet. However, some studies suggest a diet low in vitamin A, C or folate may be associated with an increased risk of cervical cancer.[4]

References

1. Parkin DM, Bray F, Ferlay J, Pisani P. Global cancer statistics, 2002. CA Cancer J Clin. 2002, 55(2): 74–108.
2. American Cancer Society. Detailed Guide: Cervical Cancer. What are the Key Statistics about Cervical Cancer? Available at: www.cancer.org. Accessed March 14, 2007.
3. Saslow D, Castle PE, Cox JT, Davey DD, Einstein MH, et al. American Cancer Society Guideline for HPV Vaccine Use to Prevent Cervical cancer and Its Precursors. CA Cancer Journal for Clinicians. 2007; 57(1):7–28.
4. Hoskins WJ, Young RC, Markman M, Perez CA, Barakat R, Randal M. Principles and Practice of Gynecologic Oncology (4th Edition). Lippincott Williams & Wilkins:Philadelphia, 2005: 634–637.
5. Villa LL. Biology of genital human papillomaviruses. International Journal of Gynecology and Obstetrics. 2006; 94(supp 1): S3–S7.
6. World Health Organization. IARC Monograph on the Evaluation of Carcinogenic Risks to Humans: Human Papillomaviruses. Vol 64. Lyons:IARC; 1995
7. Schoell WMJ, Janicek MF, Mirhashemi R. Epidemiology and Biology of Cervical Cancer. Seminars in Surgical Oncology 1999; 16:203–211.
8. Shimida T, Miyashita M, Miura S, et al. Genital human papillomavirus infection in mentally-institutionalized virgins. Gynecol Oncol 2007; Epub May 25, 2007.
9. Ley C, Bauer H, Reingold A, et al. Determinants of genital human papillomavirus infection in young women. JNCI 1991; 83:997–1003.
10. Fairley C, Chen S, Tabrizi S, et al. The absence of genital human papillomavirus infection in virginal women. Intl Journal of STD and AIDS 1992; 3:414–417.
11. Stevens-Simons C, Nelligan D, Breese P, et al. The prevalence of genital human papillomavirus infections in abused

and nonabused preadolescent girls. Pediatrics 2000; 106:654–9.

12.   Bosch FX, Qiao Y-L, Castellsague X. The epidemiology of human papillomavirus infection and its association with cervical cancer. International Journal of Gynecology and Obstetrics. 2006; 94(stpp1):S8–S21.

13.   Wright TC. Pathology of HPV infection at the cytologic and histologic levels: Basis for a 2-tiered morphologic classification system. International Journal of Gynecology and Obstetrics. 2006; 94(supp 1):S22–S31.

14.   Danso D, Lyons F, Bradbeer C. Cervical screening and management of cervical intraepithelial neoplasia in HIV-positive women. International Journal of STD & AIDS. 2006; 17(9):579–584.

15.   Denny L, Walraven S, Myer L, et al. Management of cervical disease in HIV-infected women. Gynecologic Oncology. 2005; 99(3Suppl1):S14–S15.

16.   Saraiya M, Ahmed F, Krishnan S, Richards TB, Unger ER, Lawson HW. Cervical Cancer Incidence in a Prevaccine Era in the United States, 1998-2002. Obstetrics & Gynecology. 2007; 109(2):360–370.

17.   del Carmen MG, Findley M, Muzikansky A, Roche M, Verril CL, Horowitz N, Seiden MV. Demographic, risk factor, and knowledge differences between Latinas and non-Latinas referred to colposcopy. Gynecologic Oncology. 2007; 104(1):70–76.

18.   Berrington de Gonzalez A and Green J. Comparison of risk factors for invasive squamous cell carcinoma and adenocarcinoma of the cervix: Collaborative reanalysis of individual data on 8,097 women with squamous cell carcinoma and 1,374 women with adenocarcinoma from 12 epidemiological studies. Int J Cancer. 2007, 120(4):885–91.

19.   Tsai H-T, Tsai Y-M, Yang S-F, Wu K-Y, Chuang K-Y, et al. Lifetime cigarette smoke and second-hand smoke and cervical intraepithelial neoplasm - A community-based case-control study. Gynecol Oncol 2007; 105(1):181–188.

20.   Szarewski A, Jarvis MJ, Sasieni P, et al. Effect of smoking cessation on cervical lesion size. Lancet. 1996; 347(9006):941–949.

21.   Barton SE, Maddox PH, Jenkins D, et al. Effect of cigarette smoking on cervical epithelial immunity: a mechanism for neoplastic change? Lancet 1988; 2(8612):652–4.

22.   Yasmeen S, Romano PS, Pettinger M, Johnson SR, Hubbell FA, Lane DS, Hendrix SL. Incidence of Cervical

Cytological Abnormalities With Aging in the Women's Health Initiative. Obstetrics & Gynecology. 2006; 108(2):410–419.

23. Matos A, Moutinho J, Pinto D, Medeiros R. The influence of smoking and other cofactors on the onset to cervical cancer in a southern European population. European Journal of Cancer Prevention. 2005; 14(5):485–491.

24. Stanley M. Immune responses to human papillomavirus. *Vaccine* 2006; 24(Suppl 1): S16-22.

25. Stanley M, Lowy DR, and Frazer I. Chapter 12: Prophylactic HPV Vaccines: Underlying mechanisms. *Vaccine* 2006; 24(S3):S106-13.

26. Tindle RW. Immune evasion in human papillomavirus-associated cancers. *Nat Rev Cancer* 2002; 2(1):59-65.

27. Chang YE and Laimins LA. Microarray analysis identifies interferon-inducible genes and Stat-1 as major transcriptional targets of human papillomavirus type 31. *J Virol* 2000; 74(9):4174-82.

28. Nees M, Geoghegan JM, Hyman T, Frank S, Miller, L, and Woodworth CD. Papillomavirus type 16 oncogenes downregulate expression of interferon-responsive genes and upregulate proliferation-associated and NF-kappaB-responsive genes in cervical keratinocytes. *J Virol* 2001; 75(9):4283-96.

29. Barnard P and McMillan NA. The human papillomavirus E7 oncoprotein abrogates signaling mediated by intereferon-alpha. *Virology* 1999;359(2):305-13.

30. Ronco L, Karapova AY, Vidal M, Howley PM. Human papillomavirus 16 E6 oncoprotein binds to interferon regulatory factor-3 and inhibits its transcriptional activity. *Genes Dev* 1998; 12(13):2061-72.

31. Viscidi RP, Schiffman M, Hildesheim A, Herrero R, Castle PE, Bratti MC, Rodriguez AC, Sherman ME, Wang S, Clayman B, Burk RD. Seroreactivity to human papillomavirus (HPV) types 16, 18, or 31 and risk of subsequent HPV infection: results from a population-based study in Costa Rica. *Cancer Epidemiol Biomarkers Prev.* 2004;13(2): 324-7.

32. Hildesheim A, Herrero R, Wacholder S, Rodriguez AC, Solomon D, Bratti MC,Schiller JT, Gonzalez P, Dubin G, Porras C, Jimenez SE, Lowy DR; Costa Rican HPV Vaccine Trial Group. Effect of human papillomavirus 16/18 L1 virus-like particle vaccine among young women with preexisting infection: a randomized trial. *JAMA.* 2007 Aug 15;298(7): 743-53.

CHAPTER 2

Cervical Anatomy, Histology, and Histopathology

■ Anatomy of the Cervix

- The cervix is the lower third of the uterus and projects through the upper, anterior vaginal wall (Figure 2-1).
- The size and shape of the cervix depend on several factors including age, hormonal status, and parity.
- The opening to the cervix visible in the vagina is called the external os.
- The endocervical canal is the passageway connecting the external os to the internal os, considered to be the upper limit of the cervix.
- The ectocervix is that portion of the cervix exterior to the external os.
- The cervical branches off the uterine arteries provide the blood supply to the cervix. The uterine arteries come off the internal iliac arteries.
- The nodal drainage of the cervix is complex and includes the common, internal, and external iliac nodes; the obturator; and the parametrial nodes.

■ Histology of the Normal Cervix

- The cervical epithelium gives rise to all forms of cervical precancerous and cancerous lesions.
  - It is composed of columnar and stratified squamous epithelia. The area where these meet is the squamo-columnar junction, located close to the external os.
  - Squamous epithelia are very sensitive to hormonal changes, which can induce maturation, glycogenation, and desquamation (estrogen) or inhibit them (progesterone). Changes related to human papillomavirus (HPV) infection can be seen in this layer.

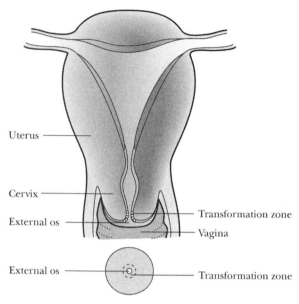

Figure 2-1: Anatomy of the cervix.

- Columnar epithelia are lined by mucus-secreting cells, and are often referred to as glandular epithelia. They line the ectocervix and the endocervical canal. Endocervical glands are formed due to the invaginations and folds that make up the endocervical canal.
- The transformation zone represents the area of metaplasia where columnar epithelia become squamous in a normal dynamic process. It is in this area that most cervical lesions develop.
- Figure 2-2 represents an example of normal epithelial cells on a Pap smear.

■ Cervical Cytopathology

- ■ Abnormal cervical findings are characterized by the *Bethesda System*.
  - It was developed in 1988 for reporting cervical or vaginal cytological diagnoses. (See Table 2-1.)

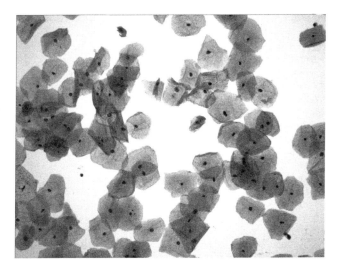

Figure 2-2: Normal Pap smear showing epithelial cells without evidence of pathologic change.

- The American Society for Colposcopy and Cervical Pathology (ASCCP) developed consensus guidelines for both diagnosis and management.[1]
- In 2001 the most recent revisions to the Bethesda System addressed statements of adequacy, general categorization, and interpretation and results of epithelial cell abnormalities.[2]
- Cervical cytopathology can be broadly classified into the following categories:
  - Atypical squamous cells (ASC)
    - Subdivided into two categories:
      - Atypical squamous cells of undetermined significance (ASC-US)
      - Atypical squamous cells, cannot exclude high-grade (ASC-H)
    - The interpretation of a cervical cytology result as ASC is poorly reproducible, even among expert pathologists.
    - Women with ASC on Pap smear may have a 5–17% chance of having a higher grade lesion

Table 2-1: The 2001 Bethesda System for Classification of Pap Smear Cytology

SPECIMEN ADEQUACY

    Satisfactory for evaluation (*note presence/absence of endocervical component*)

    Unsatisfactory for evaluation

GENERAL CATEGORIZATION *(Optional)*

    Negative for intraepithelial lesion or malignancy

    Epithelial cell abnormality

    Other

INTERPRETATION/RESULT

    Negative for Intraepithelial Lesion or Malignancy

        Organisms

        Trichomonas vaginalis

        Fungal organisms morphologically consistent with *Candida* species

        Shift in flora suggestive of bacterial vaginosis

        Bacteria morphologically consistent with *Actinomyces* species

        Cellular changes consistent with herpes simplex virus

        Other non-neoplastic findings (*Optional*)

        Reactive cellular changes associated with inflammation, radiation, etc.

        Glandular cells' status posthysterectomy

        Atrophy

    Epithelial Cell Abnormalities

        Squamous cell

            Atypical squamous cells (ASC)

                of undetermined significance (ASC-US)

                cannot exclude HSIL (ASC-H)

            Low-grade squamous intraepithelial lesion (LGSIL)

            High-grade squamous intraepithelial lesion (HGSIL)

            Squamous cell carcinoma

        Glandular cell

            Atypical glandular cells (AGC) (*specify endocervical, endometrial, or not otherwise specified*)

            Atypical glandular cells, favor neoplastic (*specify endocervical or not otherwise specified*)

            Endocervical adenocarcinoma in situ (AIS)

            Adenocarcinoma

    Other (*List not comprehensive*)

        Endometrial cells in a woman ≥40 years of age

AUTOMATED REVIEW AND ANCILLARY TESTING
(*Include as appropriate*)

*Adapted from reference 2.

on biopsy. However, in women with ASC-H, the risk of a higher grade lesion is 24–94%.
- Immunosuppressed women with ASC are at increased risk for a higher grade lesion.
- Postmenopausal women with ASC appear to be at lower risk for higher grade lesion on cervical biopsy than premenopausal women.[3]

- **Atypical glandular cells (AGC) and adenocarcinoma in situ (AIS)**
  - Subdivided into three categories:
    - Atypical glandular cells, either endocervical, endometrial, or "glandular cells" not otherwise specified (AGS NOS)
    - Atypical glandular cells, either endocervical or "glandular cells" favor neoplasia (AGS "favor neoplasia")
    - Endocervical adenocarcinoma in situ (AIS)
  - Biopsy-confirmed high-grade squamous lesions, AIS, or invasive cancer have been found in 9–41% of women with AGC NOS compared to 27–96% of women with AGS "favor neoplasia."
  - Women with cytologic interpretation of AIS have a very high risk of having either AIS (48–60%) or invasive cervical adenocarcinoma (38%).
  - Screening cervical cytology has a low sensitivity (50–72%) for detecting glandular lesions.[3]

- **Low-grade squamous intraepithelial lesion (LGSIL)**
  - Encompasses cervical intraepithelial lesions of low grade (CINI)
  - 15–30% of women with LGSIL on Pap smear will be reclassified as a higher grade lesion on cervical biopsy.
  - The majority of lesions regress without treatment.
  - HPV DNA testing does not appear to be useful for the initial management because in the ALTS study 83% of women with LGSIL were positive for high-risk HPV types.
  - The cytology of LGSIL is presented in Figure 2-3a.

(a)

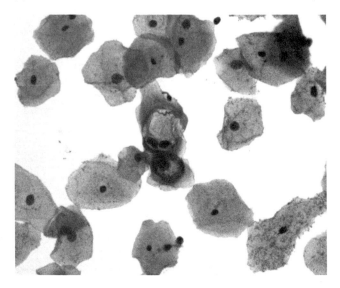

(b)

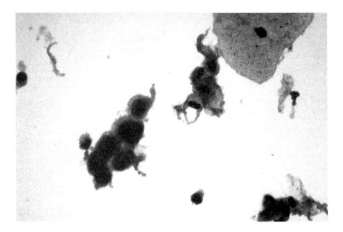

Figure 2-3: Pap smears demonstrating abnormal cytology: (a) low-grade squamous intraepithelial lesion (LGSIL); (b) high-grade squamous intraepithelial lesion (HGSIL).

- **High-grade squamous intraepithelial lesion (HGSIL)**
  - Encompasses more severe lesions, including cervical intraepithelial lesions CIN II and CIN III. It is an uncommon diagnosis, accounting for only 0.45% of cytology interpretations.
  - 1–2% chance of invasive disease.
  - The cytology of HGSIL is presented in Figure 2-3b.

■ Cervical Histopathology

- Cervical precancerous lesions have been classified in numerous ways over the years, but currently cervical intraepithelial neoplasia (CIN) classification is used. Some reduce the classifications to two entities, low-grade lesions and high-grade lesions.[3]
- **Cervical intraepithelial neoplasia classification**
  - **Low-grade lesions:**
    - **CIN I** (Figure 2-4a): Lowest-grade lesions, including condylomata.
      - May be either raised or macular.
      - Typically exhibit nuclear enlargement and hyperchromasia in the superficial epithelial cells.
      - Nuclear changes may be accompanied by koilocytotic atypia.
      - Few alterations in the lower epithelial cells.
      - Flat lesions correlate with high-risk HPV types; raised lesions correlate with low-risk HPV types.
  - **High-grade lesions:**
    - **CIN II** (Figure 2-4b): High-grade lesions.
      - Atypical cells in the lower layers of the squamous epithelium.
      - Atypical cells with changes in nucleo-cytoplasmic ratio.
      - Variation in nuclear size, loss of polarity, increased mitotic figures, and hyperchromasia.
      - Correlates strongly with high-risk HPV types.
    - **CIN III** (Figure 2-4c): High-grade lesions.

(a)

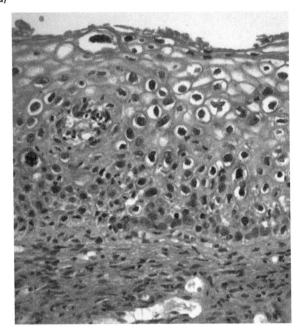

(b)

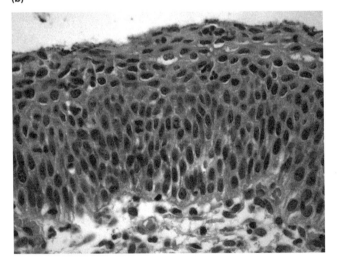

Figure 2-4: Cervical biopsy H&E staining showing cervical intraepithelial neoplasia (CIN): (a) CIN I; (b) CIN II; (c) CIN III.

(c)

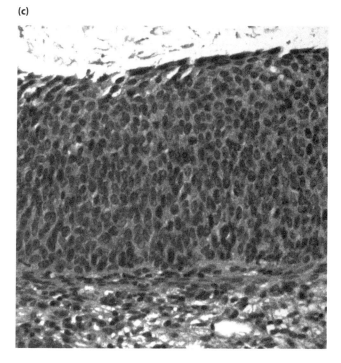

Figure 2-4: continued

- Progressive loss of differentiation.
- Greater atypia in more layers of the epithelium; no surface differentiation.
- The epithelium is totally replaced by atypical cells.
- Correlates strongly with high-risk HPV types.[3]
- Cervical carcinomas
  - Noninvasive
    - Squamous cell carcinoma in situ
      - The epithelium is replaced by atypical cells with enlarged, oval nuclei and increased nuclear to cytoplasmic ratios. Mitotic figures are present. The basement membrane is intact.
    - Adenocarcinoma in situ
      - Characterized by preservation of the overall endocervical gland architecture, but the endocervical glands and epithelium are replaced by cells

displaying atypia. Most occur near the transformation zone.

- Invasive
  - **Squamous cell carcinoma** (Figure 2-5a): (Most common) These tumors usually arise at the transformation zone. They are further classified by the following:
    - **Keratinizing:** Display at least some keratin pearl formation.
    - **Nonkeratinizing:** Composed of irregular nests of cells that may display abundant eosinophilic cytoplasm and intercellular bridges, but they do not contain keratin pearls.
    - **Verrucous:** (Rare) The cervix has papillary excrescence resembling condyloma acuminatum. Microscopically, they display papillary fronds of squamous epithelium not containing connective tissue cores.
  - **Adenocarcinoma** (Figure 2-5b): (Common) Incidence increased between the 1970s and 1990s, reaching a plateau more recently, now accounting for 20–25% of cervical carcinomas. There are a variety of types, which are described below.
    - **Endometrioid adenocarcinoma:** (Rare) Display histologic features identical to endometrial carcinoma. They have probably been overdiagnosed because of endocervical extension from the endometrium.
    - **Mucinous adenocarcinoma:**
      - Endocervical variant (Most common variant)
      - Intestinal-type, signet-ring, and colloid variants (Rare)
      - Minimal deviation variant (adenoma malignum)
      - Well-differentiated villoglandular variant
    - **Clear cell adenocarcinoma:** (Rare) Associated with diethylstilbestrol (DES) exposure.
      - The tumor has three patterns that can appear individually or together:

(a)

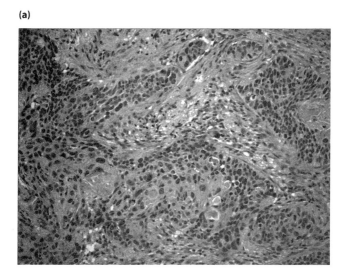

(b)

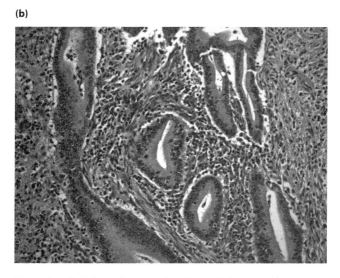

Figure 2-5: Pathology of common invasive cervical cancers: (a) squamous cell carcinoma; (b) endocervical adenocarcinoma.

- Solid pattern with sheets of cells containing glycogen-rich clear cytoplasm, atypical nuclei, and mitoses
- Tubulocystic pattern with tubules and cystic spaces lined by oxyphilic, hobnail, or clear cells
- Papillary pattern

■ **Adenosquamous carcinoma:** (Uncommon) Composed of admixed malignant glandular and squamous elements.
  - **Glassy cell carcinoma:** Very rare form of poorly differentiated adenosquamous carcinoma.
■ **Adenoid cystic carcinoma:** (Rare) Aggressive tumors
  - Cribiform gland pattern with hyaline or mucinous material
■ **Adenoid basal epithelioma:** (Rare) Indolent clinical course
■ **Small cell carcinoma:** (Rare) Most common neuroendocrine tumor seen in the cervix.
■ **Sarcomas:** (Very rare)[4]

◼ References

1. Apagar BS, Zoschnick L. The 2001 Bethesda System terminology. *Am Fam Physician*. 2003;68(10):1992–1998.
2. Solomon D, Davey D, Kurman R, et al. The 2001 Bethesda System: terminology for reporting results of cervical cytology. *JAMA*. 2002;287(16):2114–2119.
3. Wright TC, Cox JT, Massad LS, et al. 2001 Consensus guidelines for the management of women with cervical intraepithelial neoplasia. *Journal of Lower Genital Tract Disease*. 2003; 7(3):154–167.
4. Kumar V, Abba AK, Fausto N. Robbins and *Cotran Pathologic Basis of Disease (7th Ed)*. Philadelphia, PA: Elsevier, 2005.
5. Hoskins WJ, Young RC, Markman M, Perez CA, Barakat R, Randal M. *Principles and Practice of Gynecologic Oncology*. 4th ed. Philadelphia, PA: Lippincott Williams & Wilkins; 2005:634–637.

CHAPTER 3

Diagnosis and Staging

■ Screening for Cervical Pathology

- Papanicolaou (Pap) smear
  - Introduced in 1943 by Dr. Papanicolaou to detect cervical lesions.[1]
  - Between 1955 and 1992, the number of cervical cancer deaths in the United States dropped by 74%.[1] This was mainly due to the increased use of the Papanicolaou smear.
  - The conventional Pap smear has limitations, including:
    - Low sensitivity, ranging from 30% to 87%
    - High false-negative rates, ranging from 6% to 50%[2]
    - Sampling errors, with loss of up to 80% of the cellular material on the collection device
    - Interpretative limitations[3]
  - The Pap smear detects predominately precancerous cervical lesions, but occasionally will diagnose cervical cancer. Further evaluation of an abnormal Pap smear is always necessary.
- Liquid-based cytology
  - Liquid-based cytology was developed in the late 1980s in an attempt to decrease the number of false-negative Pap smears.[3]
  - There are multiple brands of liquid-based cytology.
  - Procedure
    - It is performed in the same way as a conventional Pap smear, except a plastic spatula is used.
    - The spatula and cytobrush are rinsed into a vial containing a fixative solution.
    - The slides are prepared using an automated slide processor and then removed manually and stained by the Papanicolaou method for review by pathologists.[1,3]

- With this technique, the detection rate of cytologic abnormalities is significantly increased for all cervical lesions.
- The liquid-based cytology technique had an 85% reduction in the number of times a sample was reported as less than satisfactory for cellular interpretation.[1]
- There is an increase in positive-predictive value with liquid-based cytology. Histologic follow-up of cytological reports of moderate dysplasia or greater revealed CIS, AIS, or carcinoma in 87.9% of liquid-based cytology versus 77.1% in conventional Pap smear.[3]
- The liquid-based cytology technique is thought to improve results due to the following:
  - Improved sample collection with transferal of a higher proportion of cells from the cytobrush and spatula into the vial.
  - Reduction of obscuring material because of filtration.
  - The wet fixation enhances cell preservation and nuclear morphology.[3]
- Colposcopic evaluation
  - Abnormal Pap smears are referred to colposcopy for further evaluation.
  - The exam is performed using a colposcope.
    - 3–5% ascetic acid or Lugol's solution is placed on the cervix.
    - A colposcopic exam is performed and findings are documented. See Table 3-1 for a list of colposcopic findings.[4]
  - Biopsies of the lesions are performed, along with endocervical sampling, if necessary.
  - Colposcopy with guided biopsies detects 69.9% of CIN III lesions.[5]
  - Colposcopic guided biopsies are more sensitive when two or more biopsies are taken, regardless of type or level of medical training.[5]
  - A detailed description of the treatment algorithms for abnormal Pap smears will be covered in the following chapter.

Table 3-1:   Common Coloposcopic Findings

	Acetowhite	Borders	Mosaicism	Vessels
Normal	Pale	Feathered	None	Fine/none
Low-grade lesions	Shiny gray	Distinct, jagged edges	Fine	Fine punctations
High-grade lesions	Dull oyster white	Peeling or rolled edges Internal borders	Coarse	Coarse punctations, large vessels

■ Staging

- ■ Staging systems
  - • Staging of invasive cervical cancer is derived from the International Federation of Gynecology and Obstetrics (FIGO) staging system, which is still based on clinical evaluation.[4,5] See Table 3-2.
  - • The following examinations are permitted in the FIGO staging:
    - ■ Palpation
    - ■ Inspection
    - ■ Colposcopy
    - ■ Endocervical curettage
    - ■ Hysteroscopy
    - ■ Cystoscopy
    - ■ Proctoscopy
    - ■ Intravenous urography
    - ■ Barium enema
    - ■ X-ray examination of the lungs and skeleton
    - ■ Cervical conization
  - • Compared to surgical staging, clinical staging has a high error rate, ranging from 17% to 67%.[5]
    - ■ This high error rate is likely due to the inability to identify parametrial involvement, nodal disease,

Table 3-2:   FIGO Staging for Carcinoma of the Cervix

Stage 0	Carcinoma in situ, cervical intraepithelial neoplasia, Grade 3

Stage I		Carcinoma confined to the cervix
	Ia	Invasive carcinoma diagnosed only by microscopy. Stromal invasion with a maximum depth of 5 mm and horizontal spread of <7 mm. Vascular space, venous or lymphatic, does not affect classification.
		Ia1 Measured stromal invasion 3 mm or less in depth and 7 mm or less in horizontal spread
		Ia2 Measured stromal invasion of more than 3 mm and less than 5 mm with a horizontal spread of 7 mm or less
	Ib	Clinically visible lesions limited to the cervix or microscopic lesions greater than stage Ia.
		Ib1 Clinically visible lesions less than 4 cm
		Ib2 Clinically visible lesions greater than 4 cm

Stage II		Cervical carcinoma invades beyond uterus, but not to pelvic wall or lower third of vagina
	IIa	No obvious parametrial involvement
	IIb	Obvious parametrial involvement

Stage III		The carcinoma has extended to the pelvic wall and/or involved the lower third of the vagina, and/or causes hydronephrosis or nonfunctioning kidney.
	IIIa	Tumor involves lower third of the vagina, with no extension to the pelvic wall.
	IIIb	Extension to the pelvic wall and/or hydronephrosis or nonfunctioning kidney.

Stage IV		The carcinoma has extended beyond the true pelvis or has involved (biopsy proven) the mucosa of the bladder or rectum.
	IVa	Tumor invades mucosa of the bladder or rectum, and/or extends beyond true pelvis (bullous edema is not sufficient).
	IVb	Distant metastasis

and distant metastasis, and difficulty in determining tumor size, especially if the tumor is primarily endocervical in location.

- The American Joint Committee on Cancer (AJCC) staging system uses Tumor, node, and metastases (TNM) characterization (Table 3-3); it is not used

Table 3-3:   TNM Staging of Cervical Carcinoma

Tumor Stage (T)

TX	Primary tumor cannot be assessed.
T0	No evidence of primary tumor.
T1	Cervical carcinoma confined to the uterus.
T1a1	Measured stromal invasion 3 mm or less in depth and 7 mm or less in horizontal spread.
T1a2	Measured stromal invasion more than 3 mm and not more than 5 mm with horizontal spread 7 mm or less.
T1b1	Clinically visible lesion 4 cm or less.
T1b2	Clinically visible lesion more than 4 cm.
T2	Cervical carcinoma invades beyond the uterus, but not to pelvic wall or lower third of the vagina.
T2a	Tumor without parametrial invasion.
T2b	Tumor with parametrial invasion.
T3	Tumor extends to pelvic wall and/or involves lower third of vagina, and/or causes hydronephrosis or nonfunctioning kidney.
T3a	Tumor involves lower third of vagina, no extension to pelvic wall.
T3b	Tumor extends to pelvic wall and/or causes hydronephrosis or nonfunctioning kidney.
T4	Tumor invades mucosa of bladder or rectum, and/or extends beyond true pelvis.

Nodal Staging (N)

NX	Regional lymph nodes cannot be assessed.
N0	No regional lymph node metastasis.
N1	Regional lymph node metastasis.

Distant Metastasis (M)

MX	Distant metastasis cannot be assessed.
M0	No distant metastasis.
M1	Distant metastasis.

to define stage in cervical carcinoma, but is helpful in guiding therapy in women who have undergone surgical staging. TNM staging has been proposed by the AJCC.[4]

■ Imaging

- The role of radiographic imaging in cervical carcinoma continues to evolve.

- The role of radiology has become more common in light of the invasive and expensive diagnostic procedures recommended by the FIGO guidelines. Currently these guidelines are used in less than 10% of cases.[5]
- Conventional FIGO staging methods are being replaced by computed tomography (CT) scan or magnetic resonance imaging (MRI).
  - CT and MRI can be used to better estimate the tumor size and aid in assessment of parametrial and pelvic sidewall invasion. Yet, although there is literature suggesting that use of CT and MRI is superior to clinical staging, the FIGO guidelines for routine pretreatment diagnostic evaluation have not included these imaging modalities.[8]
    - This is partially because of the belief that staging methods should be universally available. In addition, there should be a consensus on which method constitutes the most appropriate modality for women with invasive cervical cancer.[8]
  - The presence or absence of nodal metastasis has been demonstrated to be the most important prognostic factor in cervical cancer.[6]
    - CT and MRI are able to distinguish lymph nodes that are enlarged. However, these tests cannot distinguish normal-sized lymph nodes that may have metastasis. Therefore, an imaging technique that can detect normal-sized but positive lymph nodes is needed. The role of positron emission tomography (PET) is evolving in cervical cancer.[7]
  - CT scan
    - Used frequently as a single study in women with cervical cancer. When a CT scan is performed with intravenous contrast it can substitute for intravenous pyelogram to detect hydronephrosis.
    - CT scans have a sensitivity of 42% compared to a sensitivity of 29% with clinical staging in the detection of advanced stage disease.
    - In lymph nodes greater than 1 cm, sensitivity is 62.2% and specificity is 97.9%.[6]

- However, CT has a low sensitivity for detecting parametrial involvement.
- MRI
  - MRI detects 95% of cancers stage IB or higher, and is 80% accurate for evaluating depth of stromal invasion in IA tumors.
  - It has an excellent negative predictive value for stage IVA disease, whereas the FIGO staging system often underestimates bladder or rectal invasion.
  - It may be even more useful in cases of cervical adenocarcinomas, in which there is more often deep endocervical invasion.[6]
  - It has been shown to be better than CT scan or FIGO staging in the assessment of tumor size.[6]
  - However, it has similar sensitivities and specificities to CT scan in detecting nodal metastasis.
- PET scan
  - Molecular imaging technique that uses 18-fluorodeoxyglucose (FDG) to image molecular interactions of biological processes.
    - 18-FDG is not specific for malignant cells and can be noted in proliferating or inflammatory tissue.[9]
  - For invasive cervical cancer, PET is superior to CT and MRI for detecting pelvic and para-aortic lymph node metastases.[10]
    - For para-aortic node metastasis, it has a sensitivity of 75%, a specificity of 92%, a PPV of 75%, and an NPV of 92%.[9]
  - However, PET is limited in anatomic and spatial resolution.[10]
  - The role of PET scan in resectable early stage cervical cancer is unclear.
  - Some studies have suggested patients do better when followed with PET scans than if they were not, as measured by 2-year survival.[9]
  - Adding a CT scan to PET corrects the poor attenuation, localizes the lesion, and enhances the imaging quality. PET/CT can detect lesions as small as 7 mm in size.[9]

■ References

1. Solomon D, Davey D, Kurman R, et al. The 2001 Bethesda system: terminology for reporting results of cervical cytology. *JAMA*. 2002;287(16):2114–2119.

2. Guidos BJ, Selvaggi SM. Use of thin prep Pap test in clinical practice. *Diagn Cytopathol*. 1999;20(2):70–73.

3. Schledermann D, Ejersbo D, Hoelund B. Improvement of diagnostic accuracy and screening condition with liquid-based cytology. *Diagn Cytopathol*. 2006;34(11):780–785.

4. Quinn M, Benedet JL, Odicino F, Maisonneuve P, et al. Carcinoma of the cervix uteri. *Int J Gynecol Obstet*. 2006; 95(supp. 1):S43–S103.

5. Gage JC, Hanson VW, Abbey K, et al. Number of cervical biopsies and sensitivity of colposcopy. *Obstet Gynecol*. 2006; 108(2):264–272.

6. Koyama T, Tamai K, Togashi K. Staging of carcinoma of the uterine cervix and endometrium. *Eur Radiology*. 2007 Jan; [Epub ahead of print].

7. Macapinlac HA. FED-PET in the evaluation of cervical cancer. *Gynecologic Oncology*. 2005; 99(3Suppl 1):S171–2.

8. Hricak H, Gatronis C, Chi DS, et al. Role of imaging in pre-treatment evaluation of early invasive cervical cancer: results of the Intergroup Study, American College of Radiology Imaging Network 6651—Gynecologic Oncology Group 183. *J Clin Oncol*. 2005;23(36):9329–9337.

9. Lai CH, Yen TC, Chang TC. Positron emission tomography imaging for gynecologic malignancy. *Current Opinion in Obstetrics and Gynecology* 2007;19(1):37–41.

10. Choi HJ, Roh JW, Seo S-S, et al. Comparison of the accuracy of magnetic resonance imaging and positron emission tomography/computed tomography in the presurgical detection of lymph node metastases in patients with uterine cervical carcinoma. *Cancer*. 2006;106(4):914–922.

CHAPTER 4

Treatment Approaches to Preinvasive Cervical Lesions

- Cervical cancer was once a leading cause of cancer death in the United States, but now invasive cervical cancer is relatively uncommon. This shift is largely due to the increased use of cervical cytologic screening.[1]
- The introduction of screening programs in unscreened populations has been shown to reduce cervical cancer rates by up to 90% in 3 years.[2]
- Cervical cytology has been successful in decreasing the cervical cancer rates for multiple reasons, including:
  - The progression from precancerous lesions to invasive cancer is very slow, allowing ample time for dectection.
  - There are modalities for detecting cytologic and histologic abnormalities before invasive disease appears.
  - Effective and minimally invasive therapies for precancerous lesions exist.[2]
- In the United States, approximately 50 million women have Pap smears every year. Of these, approximately 7% will have a cytologic abnormality, which will need further evaluation.[3]
  - One million women will have a low-grade lesion (CIN I) and approximately 500,000 will have high-grade lesions (CIN II, III).
  - In efforts to standardize management of CIN, the American Society for Colposcopy and Cervical Pathology (ASCCP) has held consensus workshops to develop evidence-based guidelines.[1]

■ Guidelines for Management of Women with Cervical Cytological Abnormalities

Atypical Squamous Cells (ASC)

- Atypical squamous cells of undetermined significance (ASC-US)

- Repeat cervical cytological testing, colposcopy, or DNA testing for high-risk HPV are all acceptable.
- If liquid-based cytology is used or when collection for HPV DNA testing can be done, reflex HPV testing is preferred.
- DNA testing for high-risk HPV types
  - Positive: Refer for colposcopy.
  - Negative: Repeat cytology in 12 months.
- Repeat conventional or liquid-based cytology at 4- to 6-month intervals until there are two consecutive negative results.
- Women with ASC-US or greater on repeat cytology should be referred for colposcopy.
  - Normal colposcopic evaluation and biopsies: repeat cytologic examination in 12 months.
  - Confirmed CIN on biopsy: follow 2006 guidelines (see below).
- ASC-US in special circumstances
  - Postmenopausal women
    - Provide a course of intravaginal estrogen followed by a repeat cervical cytology test approximately 1 week after completion of the regimen. If repeat cytology is negative, repeat in 4 to 6 months.
    - If repeat cytology is negative again, return to annual screening.
    - If either repeat cytologic evaluation is ASC-US or greater, refer for colposcopy.
  - Immunosuppressed women
    - Referral for colposcopic evaluation.
  - Pregnant women
    - Manage the same as nonpregnant women.[3]
  - Atypical squamous cells: Cannot exclude high-grade (ASC-H)
    - Refer for colposcopic evaluation.
    - If colposcopic evaluation and biopsies are normal, then review of cytology, colposcopy, and histology results is recommended. If cytological interpretation of ASC-H is upheld, then repeat cytology at 6 and 12 months or HPV DNA testing at 12 months.

- If repeat cytology yields ASC or greater, refer for colposcopy.[3]

Atypical Glandular Cells (AGS) and Adenocarcinoma In Situ (AIS)

- Refer for colposcopic examination with endocervical sampling.
- Endometrial sampling should also be performed in all women over age 35 years and younger women with unexplained vaginal bleeding.
- Repeat cytological testing is unacceptable.
- **Atypical glandular cells, not otherwise specified (AGS NOS)**
  - Normal colposcopic exam and biopsies: repeat cytological testing at 4- to 6-month intervals until four consecutive negative results.
  - Biopsy-confirmed CIN: follow 2006 consensus guidelines (see below).
- **AGS "favor neoplasia" or AIS**
  - Proceed with colposcopic evaluation.
  - If no invasive disease is identified on colposcopic examination and cervical biopsies: perform diagnostic excisional procedure.[3]

Low-Grade Squamous Intraepithelial Lesions (LGSIL)

- Colposcopic evaluation
- If satisfactory
  - Endocervical (ECC) sampling in nonpregnant women without an identifiable cervical lesion.
  - Biopsies are negative: repeat cytological testing at 6 and 12 months or HPV DNA testing at 12 months.
  - Biopsy-confirmed CIN: Follow the 2006 consensus guidelines (below).
- If unsatisfactory
  - Endocervical sampling for nonpregnant women.
  - Biopsies are negative, ECC is negative: repeat cytological testing at 6 and 12 months or HPV DNA testing at 12 months.

- Biopsy-confirmed CIN: Follow the 2006 consensus guidelines (below).
■ Special circumstances
  - Postmenopausal women
    ■ Repeat cytological testing at 6 and 12 months with referral to colposcopy for ASC-US or greater.
    ■ HPV DNA testing at 12 months with referral for colposcopy for a positive test.
    ■ Repeat cytological testing 1 week after a course of intravaginal estrogen.
  - Adolescents
    ■ Repeat cytological testing at 6 and 12 months with referral to colposcopy for ASC or greater on repeat testing.
    ■ HPV DNA testing at 12 months with referral for colposcopy for a positive test.
  - Pregnant women
    ■ Colposcopic evaluation by experienced clinicians.
    ■ Biopsies of lesions suspicious for high-grade disease or cancer is preferred.
    ■ Biopsies of other lesions is acceptable.
    ■ *ECC is unacceptable.*
    ■ Women with unsatisfactory colposcopy should have repeat colposcopic evaluation in 6 to 12 weeks.
    ■ Reevaluation with cytology and colposcopy at least 6 weeks postpartum.[3]

High-Grade Squamous Intraepithelial Lesions (HGSIL)

■ Colposcopic evaluation with endocervical assessment.
  - If satisfactory
    ■ No lesion or only biopsy-confirmed CIN I
      - Review cytology, colposcopy, and histology results.
        ■ If remains HGSIL: diagnostic excisional procedure.
        ■ Biopsy-confirmed CIN: Follow the 2006 consensus guidelines (below).

- If unsatisfactory
    - No lesion identified
        - Review cytology, colposcopy, and histology results.
        - If remains HGSIL or CIN I: diagnostic excisional procedure.
    - Biopsy-confirmed CIN: Follow the 2006 consensus guidelines (see below).
- In women with colposcopic evaluation suggestive of a high-grade lesion, a diagnostic excisional procedure is acceptable.
- Special circumstances
    - Pregnant women
        - Colposcopic evaluation by experienced clinicians.
        - Biopsies of lesions suspicious for high-grade disease or cancer is preferred.
        - Biopsies of other lesions is acceptable.
        - *ECC is unacceptable.*
        - Women with unsatisfactory colposcopy should have repeat colposcopic evaluation in 6 to 12 weeks.
        - Unless invasive cancer is identified, treatment is unacceptable.
        - Reevaluation with cytology and colposcopy at least 6 weeks postpartum.[3]
    - Young women of reproductive age
        - Biopsy-confirmed CIN II, III is *not* identified: Observation with colposcopy and cytology at 4- to 6-month intervals for 1 year.
        - Biopsy-confirmed CIN II, III and colposcopic high-grade lesions should undergo a diagnostic excisional procedure.[3]

2006 Consensus Guidelines for the Management of Women with Cervical Intraepithelial Neoplasia

- Cervical Intraepithelial neoplasia grade 1 (CIN1)[1]
    - Preceded by ASC-US, ASC- cannot exclude HSIL, ASC-H, or LSIL cytology

- Follow-up with HPV testing every 12 months OR
- Repeat cervical cytology every 6-12 months.
  - Refer to colposcopy if HPV DNA test positive OR repeat cytology shows ASC-US or greater.
  - Return to routine cytological screening if: HPV DNA test is negative OR two consecutive repeat cytology tests are negative (for intraepithelial lesion or malignancy)
- If CIN1 persists for 2 years or more:
  - continued follow-up OR referral for excision or ablation is acceptable.
- If colposcopy is unsatisfactory, refer for diagnostic excisional procedure.
- Treatment
  - should be determined by judgment of clinician and patient values.
    - In patients with CIN1 and unsatisfactory colposcopy exam the following are considered *unacceptable*:
      - ablative procedures
      - podophyllin or podophyllin-related products for use in the vagina or on the cervix
      - hysterectomy
- Preceded by HSIL or AGC-NOS
  - Diagnostic excisional procedure OR
  - Observation with colposcopy and cytology at 6 months for 1 year
    - Both options acceptable provided that patients with AGC-NOS underwent satisfactory colposcopic examination and endocervical sampling is negative.
    - If HSIL or AGC-NOS is identified at the 6- or 12-month visit, diagnostic excision is recommended.
    - Return to routine screening if 2 consecutive results are negative for intraepithelial lesion or malignancy after 1 year.
    - If colposcopy is unsatisfactory, refer for diagnostic excisional procedure.
- Special populations:
  - Adolescent women

- Follow-up with annual cytologic assesment.
- If HSIL or greater at 12 months, refer for colposcopy.
- At 24 months, those with ASC-US or greater should undergo colposcopy.
- Follow-up with HPV DNA testing is unacceptable.
  - Pregnant women
    - Follow-up without treatment.
    - Treatment for CIN1 in this population is unacceptable.
- Cervical Intraepithelial neoplasia grade 2, 3 (CIN 2,3)[1]
  - Initial management
    - Both excision and ablation are acceptable.
    - Diagnostic excisional procedure is recommended in women with unsatisfactory colposcopy.
    - Hysterectomy is unacceptable as treatment.
  - Follow-up
    - Post-treatment management with HPV DNA testing at 6-12 months is acceptable.
    - Likewise, follow-up with cytology with or without colposcopy at 6 month intervals is also acceptable.
      - Women who are HPV DNA positive OR have ASC-US or greater at repeat cytology should undergo colposcopy with endocervical sampling.
      - Women with 2 consecutive repeat cytology tests or have a negative HPV DNA test should return to routine screening for at least 20 years starting at 12 months.
      - Repeat treatment or hysterectomy based on a positive HPV DNA test is unacceptable.
    - CIN 2,3 present at the margin of a diagnostic excisional procedure or in an endocervical sample requires reassessment with endocervical sampling at 4-6 months.
      - Proceeding to a diagnostic excisional procedure is acceptable
      - Hysterectomy is acceptable if a repeat excision is not feasible.
    - For women with recurrent or persistent CIN 2,3, a repeat diagnostic excision or hysterectomy is acceptable.

- Special populations
  - Adolescent women
    - Treatment or observation with every 6-month colposcopy and cytology for up to 24 months is acceptable, provided colposcopy is satisfactory.
    - If the appearance of the lesion at colposcopy worsens, HSIL cytology or a high-grade colposcopic lesion persists for 1 year, repeat biopsy is recommended.
    - If 2 consecutive results are negative for intraepithelial lesion or malignancy, resume routine cytological screening.
    - Treatment is recommended if CIN 3 is subsequently identified or if CIN 2,3 persists for 24 months.
  - Pregnant women
    - If the pregnancy is not in advanced stage and in the absence of invasive disease, additional colposcopic and cytological evaluation is acceptable, but done no more frequent than every 12 weeks.
    - A repeat biopsy is recommended if the lesion appearance worsens at colposcopy or if cytology suggests the presence of invasion, but deferring re-evaluation to 6 weeks or longer postpartum is acceptable.
    - Treatment in the absence of invasion is unacceptable.
    - Re-evaluation with cytology and colposcopy should not be performed within 6 weeks of delivery.
  - Adenocarcinoma in-situ (AIS)
    - IF AIS is diagnosed on an excisional procedure, then hysterectomy is the treatment of choice if women have completed child-bearing.
    - Conservative management is acceptable if future fertility is desired.
    - Re-excision is recommended if AIS is present at the margin or endometrial sampling at the time of excision showed CIN or AIS.

- reevaluation consisting of cervical cytology, HPV DNA testing, colposcopy and endocervical sampling at 6 months is acceptable.
  - Long-term follow-up is recommended if patient opts not to undergo hysterectomy.

Excisional Procedures

- Cold knife conization
  - Standard of care for treatment of CIN.
  - Removes more cervical tissue than loop excision/LEEP.
  - Is better at evaluating endocervical extension.
- Loop excision
  - Includes LEEP, large-loop excision of the transformation zone (LLETZ), and loop excision.
  - This technique uses electrocautery, which has led to some concern about thermal damage interfering with histologic assessment. However, Giacalone et al. compared histologic assessment of cold knife cone specimens versus loop excision specimens and found no difference in the sample adequacy for histologic evaluation.
  - The procedure can be performed in the outpatient setting.
  - Loop excision is as effective as traditional techniques.[4]
  - Normal histologic assessment of a LEEP specimen does not decrease the risk of recurrence.[5]
- Cryotherapy
  - Advantageous technique because it is easy to use and has a low cost.
  - Cryotherapy does not allow tailoring of treatment to the size of the lesion and does not provide a tissue specimen for histologic assessment.[6]
- Laser ablation/vaporization
  - This technique can easily be tailored to treat the exact size of the lesion.
  - The equipment required for laser ablation is very expensive and requires a moderate amount of training. In addition, this technique does not yield a tissue specimen.[6]

- Cervical conization and risk of preterm birth
  - There are conflicting data in the literature regarding the risk of preterm birth after cervical conization.
  - A recent meta-analysis found cold knife conization and LLETZ are significantly associated with preterm delivery (less than 37 weeks).[7]
  - A recent case control study found conization alone was not associated with preterm birth, but a short conization-to-pregnancy period (within 2 to 3 months) was associated with an increased risk of preterm birth.[6]

■ References

1. Wright TC Jr, Massad LS, Dunton CJ, Spitzer M, Wilkinson EJ, and Solomon D. 2006 American Society for Colposcopy and Cervical Pathology-sponsored Consensus Conference. 2006 consensus guidelines for the management of women with cervical intraepithelial neoplasia or adenocarcinoma in situ. *Am J Obstet Gynecol.* 1997;197(4):340-5.

2. Solomon D, Davey D, Kurman R, et al. The 2001 Bethesda system: terminology for reporting results of cervical cytology. *JAMA.* 2002;287(16):2114–2119.

3. Giacalone PL, Laffargue F, Aligier N, et al. Randomized study comparing two techniques of conization: Cold knife versus loop excision. *Gynecol Oncol.* 1999;75(3):356–360.

4. Livasy CA, Moore DT, Van Le L. The clinical significance of a negative loop electrosurgical cone biopsy for high-grade dysplasia. *Obstetr Gynecol.* 2004;104(2):250–254.

5. Mitchell MF, Tortolero-Luna G, Cook E, Whittaker L, Rhodes-Morris H, Silva E. A randomized clinical trial of cryotherapy, laser vaporization, and loop electrosurgical excision for treatment of squamous intraepithelial lesions of the cervix. *Obstetr Gynecol.* 1998;92(5):737–744.

6. Himes KP, Simhan H. Time from cervical conization to pregnancy and preterm birth. *Obstetr Gynecol.* 2007;109 (2,1):314–319.

7. Kyrgiou M, Koliopoulos G, Martin-Hirsch P, et al. Obstetric outcomes after conservative treatment for intraepithelial or early invasive cervical lesions: Systematic review and meta-analysis. *Lancet* 2006;367(9509):489–98.

CHAPTER 5

Treatment of Invasive Cervical Cancer

- The low incidence of cervical cancer in the United States is a testament to the value of the Pap smear as a screening test.
- With new technological advances in vaccine therapy, it may be possible to eradicate common cervical cancers, but this will not make screening obsolete.
- In the United States, most women diagnosed with cervical cancer were not screened regularly; as a result, 25% present with locally advanced disease (stage IIB through IVA).[1]
- The treatment options for early disease and locally advanced cervical cancer vary greatly.
- A summary of the treatments available surgically, medically, and with radiation oncology is given below.

■ Surgical Techniques in Cervical Cancer Therapy

- Multiple surgical techniques are employed in cervical cancer disease management, which may provide tailored surgical therapy depending on the clinical situation:
  - *Cold knife conization* is the standard of care for treatment of microinvasive cervical cancer. It does not cause thermal damage at the margins, which allows for more precise pathologic evaluation.
  - *Radical vaginal trachelectomy*
    - Developed in 1987 by Daniel Dargent. It is a modification of radical vaginal hysterectomy.
    - Involves removal of the cervix with the surrounding parametria.[7]
    - It may be an ideal option for early stage cervical cancer in young women who wish to preserve their ability to have children.

- ■ It requires an initial evaluation of lymph node basins to ensure no nodal involvement, which is considered a contraindication to trachelectomy.
- *Hysterectomy* (see Table 5-1)
  - ■ Five types of hysterectomies have been described:
    - Total (extrafascial) abdominal hysterectomy (Type I).
    - Modified radical hysterectomy (Type II) described by Ernst Wertheim more than 100 years ago.[15]
    - A radical abdominal hysterectomy with bilateral pelvic lymphadenectomy (Type III) is the most commonly performed operation for Stage IB cervical cancer; it was described by Meigs in 1944.[15]
    - Extended radical hysterectomy (Type IV) is rarely performed because it is used for tumors encroaching upon the distal ureter or parametrium, and these tumors are better treated with irradiation. However, if it is performed, the superior vesical artery is sacrificed.
    - Type V hysterectomy involves resection of a portion of the ureter or bladder.
  - ■ Complications due to radical hysterectomy are listed in Table 5-2.
- *Pelvic exenteration*
  - ■ Generally reserved for mid-line recurrences of cervical cancer.
  - ■ This procedure consists of en bloc removal of the pelvic viscera. It encompasses a radical hysterectomy, pelvic lymph node dissection, and removal of the bladder (anterior exenteration), the rectum (posterior exenteration), or both (total exenteration).[4]
  - ■ In 1948, the first case series was published on women who underwent pelvic exenteration; the mortality rate was 23%. With the addition of antibiotic therapy, intensive care monitoring, and thromboembolic prophylaxis the perioperative mortality rate has decreased to 2–14%.[11]
- *Laparoscopic techniques*
  - ■ Pelvic and para-aortic lymphadenectomy.

Table 5-1: Types of Hysterectomies Performed for Cervical Cancer

	Type I	Type II	Type III	Type IV	Type V
Vaginal cuff	Small rim removed	Proximal 1–2 cm removed	Upper one third to one half removed	Three fourths of the vagina is removed	More than one half removed
Bladder	Partially mobilized	Partially mobilized	Mobilized	Mobilized	Partially excised
Ureters	Not mobilized	Unroofed in ureteral tunnel	Completely dissected to bladder	Completely dissected to bladder and dissected from vesicouterine ligament	Partially excised
Rectum	Rectovaginal septum partially mobilized	Rectovaginal septum partially mobilized	Mobilized	Mobilized	Mobilized
Cardinal ligaments	Resected medial to ureters	Resected at level of ureter	Resected at pelvic sidewall	Resected at pelvic sidewall	Resected at pelvic sidewall
Uterosacral ligaments	Resected at level of cervix	Partially resected	Resected at post-pelvic insertion	Resected at post-pelvic insertion	Resected at post-pelvic insertion

Table 5-2: **Frequency and Complications Associated with Radical Hysterectomy**

Complication	Incidence
Early	
Urinary tract infection	9%
Fever	3.4%
Venous thrombosis	2.6%
Pulmonary thrombosis	1%
Fistulas	1.6%
Ileus	1.5%
Lymphocyst	1.6%
Ureteral obstruction	0.4%
Late	
Bladder dysfunction	2.6%
Lymphedema	3.6%
Sexual dysfunction`	2.2%

Adapted from reference 15.

- Laparoscopic radical hysterectomy (Type III) has been well described in the literature and is feasible. It is currently being performed at many institutions and has been found to be safe.
  - However, to date there have not been any randomized controlled trials comparing laparoscopic radical hysterectomy to standard therapy.[13]

■ Radiation Therapy for Cervical Cancer

- This has been used as the primary modality of treatment for cervical cancer since the 1920s.[14] The curative treatment usually includes a combination of external pelvic irradiation and brachytherapy. The cervix, paracervical tissues, and regional lymph nodes can all be encompassed in a pelvic radiation field. There are limitations to the total dose intrapelvic tissues will tolerate; bulky tumors often require larger doses to achieve locoregional control. These high doses are usually delivered with brachytherapy.[15]
  - Treatment volume

- External-beam fields are designed to include the primary tumor, paracervical tissues, and iliac and presacral lymph nodes.
- If common iliac or aortic nodes are involved, the fields are extended.
- Treatment fields are set to extend approximately 2 cm beyond the known extent of disease.
- External beam is delivered in a four-field technique to reduce the volume of tissue irradiated.
- Doses vary slightly, but most patients receive 4 to 5 weeks (45 to 50 Gy) of external therapy followed by one to two low-dose intracavitary treatments (80 to 85 Gy) or a variable number of high-dose radiation treatments.[15,16]

- Radiation dose
  - Total doses are tailored to the amount of disease at each site.
  - The Manchester system is used to specify treatment.
    - Point A: a point 2 cm lateral and 2 cm superior to the external cervical os in the plane of the implant.
    - Point B: a point 3 cm lateral to point A.
  - The total dose to point A thought to be adequate is between 75 and 90 Gy.
  - The prescribed dose for point B depends on parametrial involvement, and is between 45 and 65 Gy.[3,10,12,15]
- Complications (Table 5-3)
  - Five to fifteen percent of patients will have late complications of radiation therapy. Most gastrointestinal complications will occur within 30 months of radiation therapy. However, late complications may occur many years after treatment.[15]

■ Chemotherapy

- Though historically limited in its role for treatment of recurrent or metastatic disease, chemotherapy has assumed a much larger role in the treatment of cervical cancer, especially as part of definitive treatment for locally advanced disease in combination with radiation.

Table 5-3:   Complications Related to Radiation Therapy

Bladder:	Hematuria
	Cystitis
	Fibrosis and contraction
	Fistulas

Rectosigmoid or terminal ileum:	Bleeding
	Stricture
	Obstruction
	Perforation

Agglutination of vaginal apex

Sexual dysfunction

- Combined chemoradiation has become the standard of care as a treatment option for locally advanced cervical cancer on the basis of five positive randomized trials that prompted a National Cancer Institute Clinical Alert supporting cisplatin-based chemotherapy with radiation therapy in 1998.[24]
- A summary of the randomized controlled trials are given (also see Table 5-4):
  - Gynecologic Oncology Group (GOG) 85[18]:
    - 368 eligible patients with Stage IIB-IVA cervical cancer were randomized to receive radiation with concurrent cisplatin 50 mg/m^2 days 1 and 29, followed by 5-fluorouracil (5-FU) 1 g/m^2/day as a 96-hour infusion on days 1 and 29 versus hydroxyurea orally 2 g/m^2 twice weekly.
    - Combined cisplatin/5-FU treatment was associated with a statistically significant advantage in overall survival ($P < 0.01$), translating into a 26% reduction in the risk of death.
  - Radiation Therapy Oncology Group (RTOG) 9001[19]:
    - 403 stage IB2-IVA patients randomized to extended field radiation with cisplatin 75 mg/m^2 on days 1 and 29, followed by 5-FU 1 g/m^2/day

Table 5-4: **Summary of Randomized Trials Comparing Concurrent Chemoradiation Versus Radiation Therapy Alone in Cervical Cancer**

Trial	N (evaluable)	Therapy (All with XRT)	Survival	P-Value
GOG 85	388	Cisplatin + 5-FU Hydroxyurea	50.8% 39.8%	0.018
RTOG-9001	386	Cisplatin + 5-FU No chemotherapy	73% 58%	0.004
GOG 120	526	Cisplatin Cisplatin + 5-FU + hydroxyurea Hydroxyurea	64% 66% 39%	0.002
SWOG-8797/ GOG 109	241	Cisplatin + 5-FU No chemotherapy	81% 63%	0.01
GOG 123	369	Cisplatin No chemotherapy	84% 68%	0.008
NCIC	253	Cisplatin No chemotherapy	62% 58%	0.42

as a 96-hour infusion on days 1 and 29 versus extended field radiation alone.

- Concurrent chemotherapy with cisplatin and 5-FU was associated with a statistically significant advantage in 5-year overall survival ($P = 0.004$), translating into a 41% reduction in the risk of death.

- GOG 120[1]:
  - 526 patients stage IIB–IVA but without para-aortic node involvement were randomized to radiation concurrent with weekly cisplatin 40 mg/m^2 for 6 weeks versus cisplatin 50 mg/m^2 and 5-FU 1 g/m^2/day on days 1 and 29 given with hydroxyurea orally 2 g/m^2 twice weekly versus hydroxyurea alone.

- Both cisplatin-containing regimens showed statistically significant improvements in overall survival compared to hydroxyurea alone ($P < 0.01$) with a reduction in the risk of dying by 39–42%.
- Southwest Oncology Group (SWOG) 8797/GOG 109[20]:
  - This study randomized 241 enrolled patients with stage IB to IIA disease treated by hysterectomy, with high-risk features at final pathology defined as positive pelvic nodes, positive parametria, or positive margins.
  - Treatment was radiation alone versus chemoradiation using cisplatin 70 mg/m² on day 1 and 5-FU 1000 mg/m² on days 1–4 every 3 weeks for four cycles.
  - At 4 years, overall survival rates again favored the chemoradiation arm, 71% versus 81%, respectively ($P = 0.01$). This translated into a 51% reduction in the risk of dying.
- GOG 123[21]:
  - 369 patients with bulky stage IB disease were enrolled. Eligibility consisted of patients with an exophytic or expansile cervical lesion greater than or equal to 4 cm but without nodal involvement on CT imaging or lymphangiography.
  - Patients were randomized to radiation alone or weekly cisplatin 40 mg/m² for 6 weeks. All patients underwent a hysterectomy following treatment.
  - The pathologic complete response rate at surgery favored chemoradiation, 52%, versus radiation alone, 41%.
  - Four-year survival significantly improved in the cisplatin-arm ($P = 0.008$), translating into a 45% reduction in the risk of death.
- NCIC (National Cancer Institute of Canada) Trial[22]:
  - 259 patients with stage IB to IVA were randomized to cisplatin and radiation versus radiation alone.

- Unlike the other trials, there was no survival advantage noted at 5 years.
- Possible reasons this study failed to show a survival advantage to chemoradiation included the dosing of chemotherapy (only 70% completed full dose) and lack of standardization of radiotherapy, which varied by center.

Metastatic or Advanced Cervical Cancer

- For patients with advanced cervical cancer not amenable to surgical resection, *neoadjuvant chemotherapy* has been evaluated as a possible way to downstage tumors in order to render them operable. Although many trials have evaluated the role of neoadjuvant chemotherapy for cervical cancer, a consistent advantage in overall survival has not been demonstrated.
  - A meta-analysis of neoadjuvant chemotherapy given prior to surgery, radiation, or both treatments was performed by the Cochrane Collaboration in 2003.[23]
    - Comparing chemotherapy and radiation to radiation alone, improved survival outcomes were noted with the use of higher doses of cisplatin above 25 mg/m^2 (HR 0.91, 95% CI 0.78 to 1.05, $P = 0.20$) or shorter cycles (<14 days) (HR 0.83, 95% CI 0.69 to 1.0, $P = 0.046$).
    - Comparing the use of chemotherapy prior to surgery, radiation, or both, neoadjuvant chemotherapy was associated with a 35% reduction in the risk of death ($P = 0.0004$), though the authors acknowledged significant heterogeneity in the results and design of individual trials such that the authors could not rule out that these benefits were due to other reasons not related to neoadjuvant chemotherapy.
- Metastatic cervical cancer is not curable and treatment is palliative. Still, chemotherapy is active in this disease.
- The mainstay of therapy is cisplatin.
  - Mechanism: DNA intercalation
  - GOG 43 established 50 mg/m^2 every 3 weeks as the standard in recurrent/advanced disease with improvement in progression-free and overall survival.[24]

- Multiple trials have built on the activity of cisplatin in two- and three-drug combinations.
  - GOG 110 compared cisplatin plus mitolactol versus cisplatin plus ifosfamide versus cisplatin alone and showed a significant improvement in progression-free survival (PFS) in the cisplatin plus ifosfamide arm, without improvement in overall survival.[25]
  - GOG 149 compared cisplatin plus ifosfamide with bleomycin, ifosfamide, and cisplatin. There was no difference in PFS or overall survival.[26]
  - GOG 169 compared cisplatin plus paclitaxel with cisplatin alone. They reported an improvement in PFS, and response rates increased in the combination group from 19% to 36%. However, there was no improvement in overall survival.[27]
  - GOG 179 compared cisplatin plus topotecan with cisplatin alone. This was the first study to report a survival advantage in the combination arm compared to cisplatin alone (9.4 months versus 6.5 months). In addition, they reported improved PFS and response rates (27% versus 13%).[24]
  - Recently a Phase I/II study evaluated the toxicity and efficacy of cisplatin and gemcitabine in women with recurrent cervical cancer. They reported this combination is well tolerated and a modest response rate was seen.[28]
  - A GOG trial is currently ongoing comparing cisplatin in combination with different chemotherapeutic agents.

■ Treatment of Invasive Cervical Cancer by Stage

Early Disease

- Early invasive disease is presentation up to Stage IB.
- Stage I cervical cancer has an overall favorable prognosis with an 80% cure rate.[3]
- Poor prognostic signs (Table 5-5) include:
  - Lymph node metastases, which reduce overall 5-year survival from 82% to 90% to as low as 38%.[3]

Table 5-5: Poor Prognostic Factors for Stage IB to Stage IIA Cervical Cancer

Positive lymph node status
Primary tumor size (> 2 cm)
Depth of stromal invasion (deep 1/3)
LVSI
Parametrial extension

Adapted from references 3, 15.

- Large tumor diameter, deep stromal invasion, and lymph vascular space invasion (LVSI) were also demonstrated to predict cancer recurrence at 3 years from 2% to 31%.[3,5]
- Patients with **stage IA1** cervical cancer (defined as stromal invasion less than 3 mm in depth and horizontal extension no greater than 7 mm) have a very low risk of nodal involvement (0–4%) and can be treated conservatively.[4] However the presence of LVSI is associated with an increased risk of lymph node metastasis, in which case conservative management may not be recommended.[5] Recommended management includes:
  - Conization, which allows patients to preserve future fertility.
    - This is an acceptable treatment in women who desire future fertility, but hysterectomy remains the preferred therapy.
  - *Or* total abdominal hysterectomy
    - Abdominal, vaginal, and laparoscopic procedures are all acceptable.
  - With consideration for radiation therapy
    - Intracavitary brachytherapy alone (65 to 75 Gy to point A in one or two insertions) can be used.[4]
- For women with **Stage IA2** cervical cancer, the risk of lymph node metastasis is significantly greater than in Stage IA1. However, the number of nodes involved tends

to be lower, and thus surgery is often curative.[6] LVSI is the most important pathologic finding, indicating an increased risk of lymph node metastases, tumor recurrence, and death from disease.[6] Standard treatment recommendations include:

- Surgical management
  - Standard of care is a modified radical hysterectomy with pelvic ± (with or without para-aortic lymphadenectomy.
  - *Or* for eligible patients who wish to preserve their child-bearing potential, radical vaginal trachelectomy (Dargent's operation) with laparoscopic lymphadenectomy can be performed.[4,7]
    - Selection should be based on physician and patient preference, but the following criteria should be considered:
      - No clinical evidence of impaired fertility.
      - Lesion size <2.0 cm.
      - Limited endocervical involvement at colposcopic evaluation.
      - No evidence of pelvic node metastases.[8]
    - There have been over 100 third-trimester live births reported in the literature following radical trachelectomy.[8]
    - If attempted, nodal evaluation laparoscopically, extraperitoneally, or intra-abdominally must be performed. Positive nodal status is considered a contraindication to this procedure.
  - *Or* conization and pelvic lymphadenectomy
    - A recent retrospective study found women with tumor diameter less than 2 cm, depth of invasion less than 10 mm, negative pelvic lymph nodes, and no LVSI had only 0.63% risk of parametrial involvement. They advocate that a radical trachelectomy may be more extensive surgery than necessary in women who desire future fertility.[9] However, this procedure has not been evaluated in a randomized controlled trial to evaluate recurrence rates and overall survival.

- Radiation therapy
  - Brachytherapy alone may be used as the primary treatment.
  - In patients with positive pelvic lymph nodes, adjuvant chemoradiation with cisplatin is recommended.[10]
- For women with **Stage IB,** primary treatment may consist of radiation or radical hysterectomy with pelvic lymphadenectomy. Both have been shown to result in equivalent survival.
  - Surgical management
    - Radical hysterectomy with pelvic lymphadenectomy ($\pm$ para-aortic lymphadenectomy)
    - If lymph nodes are positive or tumor is high-risk (deep stromal invasion, positive LVSI, or involvement of surgical margins), adjuvant radiation therapy with sensitizing chemotherapy should be given postoperatively.[3,14]
  - Radiation therapy
    - Radiation therapy with sensitizing cisplatin.
- Women presenting with **Stage IB2** tumors have poorer survival rates than those presenting with earlier stage disease (70–75%). These tumors are often referred to as "bulky" or "barrel-shaped." The optimal treatment for large stage IB tumors has been controversial since the 1960s.[12]
  - The GOG performed a randomized clinical trial evaluating the role of postradiation extrafascial hysterectomy in women with bulky Stage IB cervical carcinoma. They found hysterectomy did not improve survival, but reduced the rate of local relapse.[2]
  - A subsequent GOG randomized controlled trial evaluated the benefits and risks of adjuvant pelvic radiotherapy in women with Stage IB cervical cancer treated by radical hysterectomy and pelvic lymphadenectomy. They found that the addition of radiation therapy decreased the number of local recurrences, but did not influence overall survival. However, subgroup analysis suggested that for women with bulky tumors over 4 cm in size, who had LVSI, or

who had more than one third invasion of the stroma, radiation therapy resulted in a 44% reduction in risk of recurrence.[3]

- This led to a randomized trial conducted by Keys et al. for the GOG. In this trial women with "bulky" tumors were randomized to radiation with or without weekly cisplatin concurrently. Following this, all women also underwent an extrafascial hysterectomy. This study showed improved survival rate in the group receiving combined therapy compared to radiotherapy alone, 83% versus 74%, respectively. In addition, there were fewer local recurrences and a significantly longer progression-free survival in the combined-therapy group. However, it was concluded that these improvements in survival were due to chemoradiation and not to hysterectomy.[21]

- On this basis, there are two acceptable options:
  - Radiotherapy with sensitizing cisplatin.
  - *Or* radical hysterectomy (Type III) followed by adjuvant radiotherapy and concomitant chemotherapy.

- Women with **Stage IIA** tumors are managed the same as Stage IB bulky tumors. If the tumor is felt to be respectable and the woman is a good surgical candidate, radical hysterectomy with adjuvant radiotherapy and sensitizing chemotherapy is recommended. Otherwise, the woman should be treated with radiotherapy and sensitizing chemotherapy.

Locally Advanced Disease

- **Stage IIB** to **Stage IVA** represent locally advanced disease that has extended beyond the cervix without evidence of extrapelvic extension.[16]
- Surgery is uncommon for locally advanced disease because the lateral extension of the tumor makes obtaining an adequate surgical margin unlikely.
- Chemoradiation is the standard of care for treatment of locally advanced cervical cancer.

- The use of cisplatin alone or with 5-FU with radiation therapy in locally advanced cervical carcinoma has been shown to improve survival 30–50% compared with radiation therapy alone.[17,18]
- External radiation is administered first to decrease tumor volume, and then brachytherapy is given.[16]
- The use of brachytherapy improves local control (78% versus 53%) and survival (67% versus 36%) compared to external radiation alone.[17]
- Brachytherapy has been given traditionally as low-dose-rate. However, high-dose-rate brachytherapy is becoming increasingly popular because it avoids hospitalization and prolonged patient immobilization.[16]

Advanced, Recurrent, or Persistent Disease

- Patients with **Stage IVB** disease are considered to have advanced incurable cervical cancer.
- The median 1-year survival rate for women in this group is less than 20%.[27]
- Traditionally, cisplatin has been considered the most active drug in cervical cancer. However, as cisplatin has become the mainstay of treatment of newly diagnosed cervical cancer with radiation, multiple studies have been performed evaluating platinum-based combination therapy as a means of increasing response rates and, hopefully, survival.
  - Cisplatin was compared to cisplatin plus mitolactol and to cisplatin plus ifosfamide in a GOG study. A significantly higher response rate was seen with cisplatin/ifosfamide, but no improvement in overall survival.[25]
  - Paclitaxel has a 17% response rate in advanced cervical carcinoma.[30]
  - A GOG trial compared cisplatin alone versus cisplatin plus paclitaxel in a randomized trial, and reported an improved response rate and progression-free survival. However, there was not a benefit in overall survival.[27]
  - GOG 204 is currently ongoing and is a four-arm RCT comparing cisplatin plus one of four drugs (paclitaxel, gemcitabine, topotecan, and vinorelbine).

■ Current Research in Cervical Cancer

- ■ Sentinel lymph node biopsy
  - • Lymph node status is a major prognostic factor in cervical cancer and impacts therapy. Pelvic lymph node metastases are only detected in 0–4% of Stage IA and 0–17% of Stage IB disease. This is much lower than in Stage IIA and IIB disease, where pelvic lymph node metastases occur in 12–27% and 25–39%, respectively. Therefore, lymphadenectomy may not be necessary in all patients; a search for a less invasive method has begun.[31]
  - • Sentinel lymph node dissection has been widely accepted in numerous cancers, including breast, penile, melanomas, and vulvar. However, there is little information on the feasibility and accuracy of sentinel lymph node biopsy in cervical cancer.
  - • The GOG is currently conducting a study evaluating the feasibility and accuracy of sentinel lymph node biopsy in cervical cancer.
- ■ Chemotherapy
  - • The GOG is currently performing a randomized control Phase III trial comparing cisplatin in conjunction with one of four other drugs (topotecan, vinorelbine, gemcitabine, or paclitaxel) in the treatment of Stage IVB, recurrent or persistent cervical cancer. This national phase III trial will help define the standard of care for women with advanced or metastastic cervical cancer.
  - • For women diagnosed with locally advanced cervical cancer (stage II to IVA), the GOG is performing a randomized controlled Phase III trial comparing cisplatin plus radiation versus cisplatin, tirapazamine, and radiation.

■ References

1. Rose P, Bundy B, Watkins EB, et al. Concurrent cisplatin based radiotherapy and chemotherapy for locally advanced cervical cancer. *N Engl J Med.* 1999;340(15):1144–1150.

2. Keys HM, Bundy BN, Stehman FB, et al. Radiation therapy with and without extrafascial hysterectomy for bulky stage IB cervical carcinoma: a randomized trial of the Gynecologic Oncology Group. *Gynecol Oncol.* 2003;89:343–353.

3. Sedlis A, Bundy BN, Rotman MZ, Lentz SS, Muderspach LI, Zaino RJ. A randomized trial of pelvic radiation therapy versus no further therapy in selected patients with stage IB carcinoma of the cervix after radical hysterectomy and pelvic lymphadenectomy: a Gynecologic Oncology Group study. *Gynecol Oncol.* 1999;73:177–183.

4. Hoskins WJ, Young RC, Markman M, Perez CA, Barakat R, Randal M. Principles and Practice of Gynecolgic Oncology. (4th Edition). Lippincott Williams & Wilkins; 2005:634–637.

5. Sevin BU. Management of Microinvasive Cervical Cancers. Seminars in Surgical Oncology 1999; 16(3): 228–231.

6. Buckley SL, Tritz DM, Van Le L, Higgins R, Sevin B-U, et al. Lymph Node Metastases and Prognosis in Patients with Stage IA2 Cervical Cancer. Gynecologic Oncology 1996; 63(1):4–9.

7. Dursun P, LeBlanc E, Nogueira MC. Radical vaginal trachelectomy (Dargent's operation): a critical review of the literature. *Eur J Surg Oncol.* 2007 Jan; [Epub ahead of time]

8. Burnett AF. Radical trachelectomy with laparoscopic lymphadenectomy: review of oncologic and obstetrical outcomes. Current Opinion in Obstetrics and Gynecology 2006; 18(1):8–13.

9. Stegeman M, Louwen M, van der Velden J, et al. The incidence of parametrial tumor involvement in select patients with early cervix cancer is too low to justify parametrectomy. Gynecologic Oncology 2007; 105(2)475–80.

10. Peter WA, Liu PY, Barrett RJ, et al. Concurrent chemotherapy and pelvic radiation therapy compared with pelvic radiation therapy alone as adjuvant therapy after radical surgery in high-risk early-stage cancer of the cervix. *J Clin Oncol.* 2000;18(8):1606–1613.

11. Marnitz S, Kohler C, Muller M, Behrens K, Hasenbein K, Schneider A. Indications for primary and secondary exenterations in patients with cervical cancer. Gynecologic Oncology 2006;103(3):1023–1030.

12. Keys HM, Bundy BN, Stehman FB, et al. Cisplatin, radiation, and adjuvant hysterectomy compared with radiation and adjuvant hysterectomy for bulky stage IB cervical carcinoma. *N Engl J Med.* 1999;340(15):1154–1161.

13. Spiritos NM, Eisenkop SM, Schlaerth JB, Ballon SC. Laparoscopic radical hysterectomy (type III) with aortic and pelvic lymphadenectomy in patients with stage I cervical cancer: Surgical morbidity and intermediate follow-up. Am J Obstet Gynecol 2002;187(2):340–348.

14. Novetsky AP, Einstein MH, Goldberg GL, Hailpern SM, et al. Efficacy and toxicity of concomitant cisplatin with external beam pelvic radiotherapy and two high-dose-rate brachytherapy insertions for the treatment of locally advanced cervical cancer. *Gynecol Oncol.* 2007 Feb; [Epub ahead of print].

15. Berek JS, Hacker NF. *Practical gynecologic oncology.* 4th ed.: Philadelphia, PA: Lippincott Williams & Wilkins; 2005: 337–396.

16. Rose PG. Stage IIB–IVA cancer of the cervix. *Cancer J.* 2003;9(5):404–414.

17. Komaki R, Brickner TJ, Hanlon AL, et al. Long-term results of treatment of cervical carcinoma in the United States in 1973, 1978, and 1983. Patterns of Care Study (PCS). *Int J Radiat Oncol Biol Phys.* 1995;31(4):973–982.

18. Whitney CW, Sause W. Bundy BN, et al. A randomized comparison of fluorouracil plus cisplatin versus hydroxyurea as an adjunct to radiation therapy in stages IIB-IVA carcinoma of the cervix with negative para-aortic lymph nodes. A Gynecologic Oncology Group and Southwest Oncology Group study. *J Clin Oncol.* 1999;17(5):1339–1348.

19. Morris M, Eifel PJ, Lu J, et al. Pelvic radiation with concurrent chemotherapy compared with pelvic and para-aortic radiation of high-risk cervical cancer. *N Engl J Med.* 1999; 340(15):1137–1143.

20. Peters WA 3rd, Liu PY, Barrett RJ 2nd, et al. Concurrent chemotherapy and pelvic radiation therapy compared with pelvic radiation therapy alone as adjuvant therapy after radical surgery in high-risk early-stage cancer of the cervix. *J Clin Oncol.* 2000;18(8):1606–1613.

21. Keys HM, Bundy BN, Stehman FB, et al. Cisplatin, radiation, and adjuvant hysterectomy compared with radiation and adjuvant hysterectomy for bulky stage IB cervical carcinoma. *N Engl J Med.* 1999;340(15):1154–1161.

22. Pearcey R, Brundage M, Drouin P, et al. Phase III trial comparing radical radiotherapy with and without cisplatin 40 mg/m^2 weekly for 5 weeks in patients with advanced squamous cell cancer of the cervix. *J Clin Oncol.* 2002; 20(4): 966–972.

23. Neoadjuvant Chemotherapy for Cervical Cancer Meta-Analysis Collaboration (NACCCMA). Neoadjuvant chemotherapy for locally advanced cervical cancer. *Cochrane Database Systematic Reviews.* 2004;2:CD001774.

24. Long HJ, Bundy BN, Grendys EC, et al. Randomized phase III trial of cisplatin with or without topotecan in carcinoma of the uterine cervix: a Gynecologic Oncology Group study. *J Clin Oncol.* 2005;23(21):4626–4633.

25. Omura GA, Blessing JA, Vaccarella L, et al. Randomized trial of cisplatin versus cisplatin plus mitolactol versus cisplatin plus ifosfamide in advanced squamous carcinoma of the cervix: A Gynecologic Oncology Group study. *J Clin Oncol.* 1997;15(1):165–171.

26. Buxton E, Meanwell C, Hilton C, et al. Combination bleomycin, ifosfamide, and cisplatin chemotherapy in cervical cancer. *J Natl Cancer Inst.* 1989;81(5):359–361.

27. Moore DH, Blessing JA, McQuellon RP, et al. Phase III study of cisplatin with or without paclitaxel in stage IVB, recurrent, or persistent squamous cell carcinoma of the cervix: a Gynecologic Oncology Group study. *J Clin Oncol.* 2004;22 (15):3113–3119.

28. Matulonis UA, Campos S, Duska L, Krasner CN, et al. Phase I/II dose finding study of combination cisplatin and gemcitabine in patients with recurrent cervix cancer. *Gynecol Oncol.* 2006; 103(1):160–164.

29. Rose PG. Concurrent chemoradiation for locally advanced carcinoma of the cervix: where are we in 2006? *Ann Oncol.* 2006;17(suppl. 10):224–229.

30. McGuire WP, Blessing JA, Moore DH, et al. Paclitaxel has moderate activity in squamous cervix cancer: A Gynecologic Oncology Group study. *J Clin Oncol.* 1996; 14(3):792–795.

31. Barranger E, Coutant C, Cortez A, Uzan S, Darai E. Sentinel node biopsy is reliable in early-stage cervical cancer but not in locally advanced disease. *Ann Oncol.* 2005;16(8): 1237–1242.

Prevention and Screening

- Cervical cancer is an inherently treatable and curable disease if caught early.
- Pap smears are among the most successful screening tests in use, and its more widespread use has dramatically reduced the incidence and deaths from invasive cervical cancer.
- In addition to screening, decreasing risks should be emphasized and newer technologies utilized.

■ American Cancer Society Guidelines for Cervical Cancer Screening

- Cervical cancer screening should begin approximately 3 years after the onset of vaginal intercourse, but no later than 21 years of age.
  - This recommendation is based on the natural history of HPV infection and of cervical lesions. There is very little risk of missing an important cervical lesion until 3 to 5 years after initial exposure to HPV.
  - There is concern that screening before the suggested 3 years may result in overdiagnosis of cervical lesions that will regress spontaneously.
  - The upper age limit for when to initiate screening is for providers who do not ask for a sexual history or adolescents who do not disclose a history of intercourse.
  - In women with HIV, a Pap test should be performed twice the first year after diagnosis and annually thereafter.
- Women who are age 70 and older, with an intact cervix and a history of three documented, consecutive, satisfactory negative cervical cytology tests and no abnormal tests within the previous 10 years may cease screening.

- The age 70 is somewhat arbitrary and other organizations choose 65 years of age. Cervical cancer is rare among older screened women, and it becomes more difficult to obtain satisfactory samples secondary to atrophy and cervical stenosis in older women.
- Women who have had a hysterectomy for benign disease and had a history of normal cervical cytology testing prior to hysterectomy do not need to continue with vaginal cytology testing.
  - Women with a history of exposure to DES or a subtotal hysterectomy should continue screening.
  - For women with a history of CIN II/III, follow-up cytology should be performed every 4 to 6 months until three documented negative vaginal cytology tests.
- Cervical screening should be performed annually with conventional cervical cytology and every 2 years with liquid-based cytology. At age 30, women with three consecutive negative cytology results and a negative test for high-risk HPV may be screened every 2 to 3 years.
  - If women have been exposed to DES in utero, are HIV+, or are immunocompromised, they should continue annual screening.
- Women age 30 and over may have cervical cytology testing with HPV DNA testing.
  - If the cytology and high-risk HPV are both negative, they should not be rescreened before 3 years.[1,2]
  - If the results are negative by cytology, but they are high-risk HPV DNA positive, repeat HPV DNA testing along with cervical cytology in 6 to 12 months should be performed. If either result is abnormal, colposcopy should be performed.[2]

■ Preventing Cervical Cancer: HPV Vaccination

- HPV is the most common sexually transmitted infection.
- In the United States, over 6 million people are infected with genital HPV each year, and approximately 15% of the population is currently infected.
- Virtually all cervical cancers are related to HPV, and approximately 70% are caused by HPV types 16 or 18.[3]

- Although the vast majority of HPV infections do not result in cervical cancer, it is clear that persistence of HPV infection carries with it a risk of developing the disease.
- Prevention requires reduction in risk behaviors that could predispose one to this and other sexually transmitted diseases. However, the protective effects of condoms are unknown.
- Breakthroughs in vaccine therapy have been developed that may help make cervical cancer the first malignancy to be eradicated.
- Table 6-1 gives the American Cancer Society's recommendations for vaccination against HPV.
- Two prophylactic HPV vaccines have been developed; they are compared in Table 6-2. Both are subunit vaccines, based on the finding that the major capsid protein of HPV, L1, self-assembles into virus-like particles (VLP) that resemble the outer shell of HPV and induce high titers of antibodies that neutralize virions.[4]
- Trials evaluating vaccination in male populations are ongoing. Researchers are evaluating these strategies in HIV-positive and negative men, including both heterosexual men, and men who have sex with men (MSM). To date,

Table 6-1:   ACS Recommendations for HPV Vaccine Use

- Routine HPV vaccination is recommended for females ages 11 to 12 years.

- Females as young as age 9 years may receive HPV vaccination.

- HPV vaccination is also recommended for females ages 13 to 18 years.

- A decision about whether women ages 19 to 26 years should receive the vaccine should be based on an informed discussion with each woman and her health care provider.

- HPV vaccination is not recommended for women over age 26 or males.

- Cervical cytology screening should continue in vaccinated and unvaccinated women.

Table 6-2:   Prophylactic Vaccines Against HPV

	Quad HDV 16/18/6/11	Bivalent + HPV 16/18 ASO4 Ajuvanted
Manufacturer	Merck	GlaxoSmithKline
Type	Tetravalent	Bivalent
HPV-strain VLPs*	6, 11, 16, 18	16, 18
Adjuvant used	Aluminum phosphate	ASO4 (aluminum salt plus monophosphoryl lipid A)
Production	*Saccharomyces cerevisiae* (yeast)	Recombinant-baculovirus infected cells
FDA indications	Prophylaxis against cervical cancer and against cutaneous genital warts	Filed for US approval, March 2007
Vaccination schedule	3 injections at 0, 2, and 6 months	3 injections at 0, 1, and 6 months
Efficacy:		90%
- protection against infection	100%	
- protection against CIN2+ lesions	98%	
Cross Protection	31, 33, 35, 39, 45 51, 52, 56, 58, 59[15]	31, 33, 35, 39, 45, 51, 52, 56, 58, 59, 66, 68[16]

*VLP: virus-like particles.

however, there is no data on the effectiveness of vaccination in boys or men, and they remain areas of active investigation.

Quad HDV 16/18/6/11

- FDA approved for prevention of cervical cancer and other diseases in females caused by HPV.
  - Tetravalent vaccine containing VLPs of HPV 6, 11, 16, and 18.

- HPV 6 and 11 are nononcogenic but are the major causative virus of cutaneous genital warts.[4]
■ Indicated as *prophylaxis,* prior to infection with HPV, not after infection has been established.
■ Quad HDV 16/18/6/11 efficacy has been established in clinical trials:
  - Koutsky et al. first reported results of a univalent vaccine using HPV-16 VLP.[5] Eligible patients were between 16 and 23 years old with less than five male partners during their lifetime. Vaccine versus placebo was administered at 0, 2, and 6 months. Results at a median follow-up of 3.5 years were published separately.[6] The vaccine afforded 94% effectiveness with 7 patients with persistent HPV-16 infection versus 111 patients receiving placebo. It was 100% effective in the prevention of CIN I (0 cases in vaccinated patients versus 24 cases in placebo group).
  - The tetravalent vaccine was evaluated in an international trial and results published.[7] In a study involving over 450 patients, the vaccine induced 90% protection against persistent HPV infection and 100% protection against CIN I. Follow-up in a subset of 241 patients showed that the efficacy of vaccination was sustained through 5 years of follow-up.[8]
  - Pooled analyses from randomized trials were presented at the 2007 AACR meeting in which data involving over 12,000 women between 16 and 23 years old were randomized to vaccine or placebo and followed through 3 years after vaccination.[8] In those women completing protocol therapy, vaccine efficacy was 98% against HPV 16- or 18-related CIN and AIS.
  - A pre-planned subgroup analysis of over 9000 women treated on trials comparing Quad HDV 16/18/6/11 versus placebo evaluated the cross-protection against HPV strains beyond those included in the tetravalent vaccine. They showed

that vaccination reduced the risk of infection by ten other oncological HPV types by 38%.[15]

- Current trials using population-based cohorts are ongoing to establish the long-term efficacy of vaccination using Quad HDV 16/18/6/11.[10]

■ The major side effects of immunization were mild or moderate local reactions after injection.

■ Despite vaccination, routine and regular Pap screening is still required because women will still be at risk for infection from other HPV types, which could also cause cervical cancer.

Bivalent + HPV 16/18 ASO4 Ajuvanted

■ Filed for FDA approval in March 2007.

■ The vaccine is formulated with a proprietary immune booster called ASO4 adjuvant, composed of aluminum salt plus monophophoryl lipid A.[4] Vaccines with novel adjuvants may afford stronger, more robust, and more sustained immune responses. Gianni et al. reported higher and more sustained antibody responses (1.6 to 4.1-fold) when a vaccine contained the novel ASO4 adjuvant, compared to adjuvant aluminum hydroxide.

■ It requires three vaccinations over a 6-month period.

■ An extended follow-up study of over 700 women between the ages of 15 and 25, and treated in the randomized clinical trial of Bivalent + HPV 16/18 ASO4 Ajuvanted or placebo, showed that immunization was sustained up to 5.5 years. In addition, cross-protection against HPV stains 45 and 31, which were not included in the vaccine preparation, was also noted.[12,13]

- However, for both vaccines there is little information currently available on the duration of HPV vaccine-induced immunity and whether booster immunizations will be required.

- The interim results of an international phase III trial involving 18,664 women aged 15-25 years old was recently published.* In this study women were randomly given the HPV 16/18 vaccine or hepatitis A vaccine at 0, 1, and 6 months. With a median follow-up of 15 months, there were 2 cases of CIN2 in the group who received the HPV vaccine, versus 21 in the group receiving Hepatitis A vaccine. The efficacy against CIN2+ disease that was HPV 16/18 DNA positive was 90.4% (p < 0.0001). Cross-protection was also demonstrated (see Table 6-2).

- Implications for vaccination
  - Despite cervical cancer declines in the United States, it remains a worldwide issue, particularly in the developing world.
  - If worldwide vaccination does lead to long-lasting immunity, it can potentially reduce the incidence of HPV infection and, hence, reduce the rates of diagnosis and ultimately deaths related to cervical cancer.
  - Even within the United States, it may lead to fewer abnormal Pap smears, which could result in reduction in medical costs by decreasing the number of biopsies, invasive procedures, and repeat tests required.
  - VLP vaccines are not expected to induce regression of established HPV-induced neoplasia.
  - The current vaccines have limitations from a worldwide prospective.
    - They are expensive to manufacture.
    - They are expensive to distribute because they involve intramuscular injection that requires a cold chain for storage.
    - Protection may be predominately type-specific and may not protect against almost 30% of cervical cancers. In developing countries that do not have effective screening programs, vaccination may provide hope in controlling the incidence of cervical cancer. It should also induce a strong immune response, which is sustainable into the future.
  - An ideal HPV vaccine would be inexpensive, protect against all oncogenic types, require a single vaccination. Development of second-generation vaccines and other prevention strategies are under way.[14]

■ References

1. Saslow D, Runowicz CD, Solomon D, et al. American Cancer Society guidelines for the early detection of cervical neoplasia and cancer. *J Lower Genital Tract Dis.* 2003;7(2): 67–86.

2. Wright TC, Schiffman M, Solomon D, et al. Interim guidance for the use of human papillomavirus DNA testing as an adjunct to cervical cytology screening. *Obstet Gynecol.* 2004; 103(2):304–309.

3. Saslow D, Castle PE, Cox TJ, et al. American Cancer Society Guideline for Human Papillomavirus (HPV) Vaccine Use to Prevent Cervical Cancer and Its Precursors. *CA Cancer J Clin.* 2007;57(1):7–28.

4. JT Schiller and DR Lowy. Prospects for cervical cancer prevention by human papillomavirus vaccination. *Cancer Res.* 2006; 66(21):10229–32.

5. LA Koutsky, KA Ault, CM Wheeler, et al. A controlled trial of a human papillomavirus type 16 vaccine. *NEJM* 2002; 347(21):1645–51.

6. C Mao,LA Koutsky, KA Ault, et al. Efficacy of human papillomavirus-16 vaccine to prevent cervical intraepithelial neoplasia: a randomized controlled trial. *Obstet Gynecol* 2006; 107(1):18–27.

7. LL Villa, RL Costa, CA Petta, et al. Prophylactic quadrivalent human papillomavirus (types 6, 11, 16, and 18) L1 virus-like particle vaccine in young women: a randomized double-blind placebo-controlled multicentre phase II efficacy trial. *Lancet Oncol.* 2005; 6(5):271–8.

8. LL Villa, RL Costa, CA Petta, et al. High sustained efficacy of a prophylactic quadrivalent human papillomavirus types 6/11/16/18 virus-like particle vaccine through 5 years of follow-up. *Br J Cancer* 2006; 95(11):1459–66.

9. D. Brown High sustained efficacy of a prophylactic quadrivalent human papillomavirus (HPV) (Types 6, 11, 16, 18) L1 virus-like particle (VLP) vaccine against cervical intraepithelial neoplasia (CIN) grades 2/3 and adenocarcinoma in situ (AIS). Presented at the American Assoc of Cancer Res Annual Meeting. April 17, 2007, Los Angeles, CA.

10. M Lehtinen, D Apter, G Dubin, et al. Enrollment of 22,000 adolescent women to cancer registry follow-up for long-term human papillomavirus vaccine efficacy: guarding against guessing. *Int J STD AIDS.* 2006; 17(8):517–21.

11. Giannini SL, et al. Superior immune response induced by vaccination with HPV 16/18 L1 VLP formulated with AS04 compared to aluminum salt only formulation. The 4th Annual International Conference on Frontiers in Cancer Prevention Research (AACR); October 2005; Baltimore, MD, Poster B68.

12. Harper DM, Franco EL, Wheeler C, et al. Efficacy of a bivalent L1 virus-like particle vaccine in prevention of infection with human papillomavirus types 16 and 18 in young women: a randomised controlled trial. *Lancet.* 2004;364 (9447):1757–65.

13. Gail SA, Teixera J, Wheeler CM, et al. Substantial impact on precancerous lesions and HPV infections through 5.5 years in women vaccinated with the HPV-16/18 L1 VLP ASO4 candidate vaccine. Paper presented at the American Association of Cancer Research Annual Meeting; April 2007; Los Angeles, CA.

14. Schiller JT, Nardelli-Haefliger D. Chapter 17: second generation HPV vaccines to prevent cervical cancer. *Vaccine.* 2006;24(suppl. 3):147–153.

15. Brown DR. HPV Type 6/11/16/18 Vaccine: First Analysis of Cross-Protection against Persistent Infection, Cervical Intraepithelial Neoplasia (CIN), and Adenocarcinoma In Situ (AIS) Caused by Oncogenic HPV Types in Addition to 16/18. Abstract G-1720b: 47th Interscience Conference on Antimicrobial Agents and Chemotherapy, Sept.17-20, 2007.

16. Paavonen J, Jenkins D, Bosch FX, Naud P, Salmerón J, Wheeler CM, Chow SN, Apter DL, Kitchener HC, Castellsague X, de Carvalho NS, Skinner SR, Harper DM, Hedrick JA, Jaisamrarn U, Limson GA, Dionne M, Quint W, Spiessens B, Peeters P, Struyf F, Wieting SL, Lehtinen MO, and Dubin G. HPV PATRICIA study group. Efficacy of a prophylactic adjuvanted bivalent L1 virus-like-particle vaccine against infection with human papillomavirus types 16 and 18 in young women: an interim analysis of a phase III double-blind, randomised controlled trial. Lancet. 2007 Jun 30;369(9580):2161-70.

Index

Note: The *f* or *t* following page numbers indicate figures or tables, respectively